Finding Home
Journal
THE COMPANION GUIDE

Finding Home

Journal

THE COMPANION GUIDE

MAHNAZ JAHANGIRI

Finding Home Journal: The Companion Guide
Published by Mahnaz Jahangiri
Thousand Oaks, California

Jahangiri, Mahnaz
Finding Home
Mahnaz Jahangiri

ISBN: 979-8-9861592-2-5, 979-8-9861592-4-9 Journal Book

Finding Home: A Path to Emotional Stability and Self Healing (2nd Edition)
ISBN: 979-8-9861592-0-1, 979-8-9861592-3-2 Paperback
ISBN: 979-8-9861592-1-8 Digital

Self-Help / Journaling
Body, Mind & Spirit > Healing > Prayer & Spiritual
Health & Fitness > Yoga

Photographs by Heirlume Photography.
Book design by Michelle M. White.

QUANTITY PURCHASES:
Schools, companies, professional groups, clubs, and other organizations
may qualify for special terms when ordering quantities of this title.
For information, email info@samadiyoga.com.

Samadi Yoga

"Go within. Use the inner body as a starting point
for going deeper and taking your attention
away from where it's lodged, in the thinking mind."

~ Eckhart Tolle

Contents

Welcome

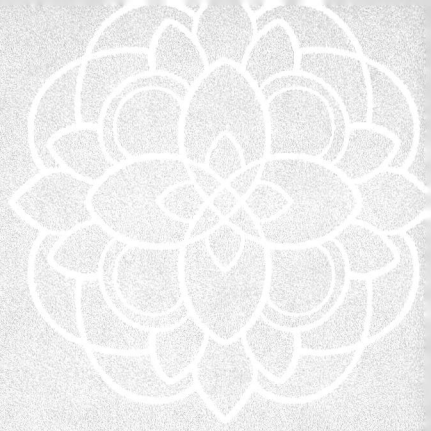

Welcome to your 12-month journey on creating a path for optimal health — mentally, emotionally, physically, and spiritually. This journal serves as a companion guide to my book, *Finding Home: A Path to Emotional Stability and Self-Healing*.

A common theme you may encounter during your journey is "recognition". Through the self-observations, self-reflections, and consistent practice of yoga and meditation, you may begin to *recognize* certain thoughts, habits, and behaviors within yourself. The dive into deeper self-understanding will help you become clearer and more in-tune with your inner workings. My wish for you is to become the observer and not the judge of habits that may be holding you back. With guidelines, self-reflection questions and practices, I wish for you to implement habits that help uplift and support you to the highest levels of well-being along with a deeper connection to Self.

The chapter topics in this journal coincide with the chapters in *Finding Home - Second Edition*. You may progress through the journal one chapter per month or every four weeks.

At the end of each chapter, you will find 5 blank weekly Wellness Calendars. These calendars help you organize and plan your practice for the month. This way, the weekly program is a commitment and implementation based on your individual schedule.

Also provided are four different yoga practice sequences that progressively build upon the preceding sequence. Each are written in step-by-step format along with an option to view a live video using QR codes. You will also be provided with helpful tips for building your own meditation practice, which can also be scheduled in your Wellness Calendar. The meditation sessions are encouraged in addition to the physical yoga practices. Collectively, the yoga and meditation practices — along with self-reflection questions — guide you towards improved physical, mental, and emotional health, overall calm, and well-being, and in time, lead you to a consistently deeper connection to Self.

HOW TO USE YOUR JOURNAL

Each month leads you through *self-reflection journaling* based on the chapter's topics. Journaling boosts our health by helping us process emotions, deepen our self-discovery, and increase well-being by reducing stress.

Self-reflection Journaling

The self-reflection questions in many of the chapters are designed for you to contemplate your personal experiences as they relate to each topic. The exercises help you further understand and observe your internal world and internal processes.

Journaling helps us manage the emotions by helping *name* what we are feeling. Once we name it, we can work with the challenge honestly within ourselves. It forces us to use words to describe what we are internalizing. The act of writing helps us identify the outcome by labeling it, expressing the effect of the challenge on our emotions so we can acknowledge and mentally organize it. This way, we have a better chance of moving past the difficulty and continuing forward. Journaling serves to decrease our worries and distractions by increasing our mental capacity and memory. We tend to obsess less about the challenge, thought or emotion when we put pen to paper — literally and figuratively — and in turn, we are inclined to resist less. Sometimes our resistance to the difficulty is a bigger test than the challenge itself.

In addition to journal pages to write in, you'll find your Wellness Calendar to schedule and increasingly build meditation and yoga practices into your daily life.

Wellness Calendars

Using the *weekly calendars,* map out your ideal practice times including the *days of the week* and *times of day*. Write down the days you will practice yoga and meditation at the start of each week and do your best to commit to it. Each month you are given guidelines for the number of days per week you aim to practice.

There are 4 sequences in this journal. Each sequence can be used for the subsequent 3 months. The first sequence is designed to be used for months 1–3, the second sequence is designed to be used for months 4–6, the third sequence for months 7–9, and the last sequence for months 10–12. Based on your progress and allotted time, each sequence can be done as a complete class or practiced in 2 sessions. The first half of the class can be done as one session and the 2nd half can be done as another session.

The blank weekly calendars are organized into five columns. Each column helps you create your personal wellness plan. The first column lists the days of the week where you schedule your practices. The second column is the *Niyama* column, where you schedule the activities you enjoy. The third column is the *Asana* column, where you write the intended physical practice and duration, such as a 20-minute floor or standing sequence, or the style such as Hatha or Vinyasa. The fourth column is for *Meditation,* where you write down the duration of each session. The last column is *Observations,* where you *highlight changes* in the body in the physical yoga practices or your experiences during your meditation sessions.

Ideally, make notes on both. This calendar helps create consistency, brings awareness to your practices, and reinforces self-discovery in both mind and body.

Niyama Column

This portion of the calendar is for you to schedule weekly activities that bring you joy. Niyama is a Sanskrit term and the 2nd limb of yoga philosophy that means treating ourselves with respect, love, and compassion, and taking care of our own mental, emotional, and physical well-being.

The *Niyama* column is for you to plan activities that you enjoy and make them part of your weekly *Wellness Calendar*. The activities can range from taking time to read your favorite book, get a massage, or spend time in nature. Pausing to simply enjoy activities you love helps reinforce a sense of balance and calm. Soon you notice these practices become part of your weekly routine.

Asana Column

Asana is a Sanskrit term and the 3rd limb of yoga philosophy that means the physical practice of conditioning the body. The *Asana* column is designed for you to write down the duration and format of your practice. You may write down a 20- or 40-minute practice. You may also note whether you schedule a floor or standing sequence or even a Hatha or Vinyasa style sequence. You are encouraged to write your experiences of each practice under the "Observations" column.

Meditation Column

Meditation practices are more challenging than physical practices. The physical practice of yoga or "Hatha" blossomed to prepare the body for the more advanced yoga practices of meditation and insight. Since meditation is challenging, start out in smaller increments and build up your practice. Keep track by writing down how long each session is or lasts. You may log the varying fluctuations of the mind on each given session under the "Observations" column. In Chapter 2 of this journal, you will find tips for meditation practice along with a QR code for a live video recording sharing more tips and practices!

Beginning Meditation Guidelines for Month #1

1. Set a timer for 1- 3 minutes

2. Sit comfortably in an upright position and be still.

3. Focus on the Breath.

    Observe the inhale and exhale (Avoid manipulating the breath and feel the flow of each inhale and exhale as it is.)

Observations

Observations are another important aspect of creating effective practices. On each day you practice Physical Yoga or Asana, write down a few lines about how the body felt and responded. You may notate the energy levels in the body, the varying amounts of strength, changes in flexibility and mobility, or the level of progress in a particular pose. Keep in mind that each day the body is different. The body responds to varying sleep patterns, food intake, weather, stress levels, and emotions. Take time to observe and reflect on your discoveries after each practice. Writing your observations helps bring attention to the subtle changes while reinforcing bodily awareness.

In addition, write down your observations for each meditation sitting. This practice of observing, reflecting, and documenting each experience helps you pay more attention to mental fluctuations. Making note of each meditation practice reinforces the "observer" approach rather than the identifier. When we observe, we create space for clarity, yet when we identify, we limit ourselves in judgment and healing. Writing mental and emotional observations reinforces self-awareness.

Yoga Sequences

The *yoga sequences* are outlined step-by-step and are also available in video format on the **Samadi Yoga** website. You can access the videos using the QR codes, which conveniently direct you to each sequence on the website.

To use the QR codes on your compatible smartphone or tablet, open the built-in camera app. Point the camera at the QR code. Tap the banner that appears on your phone or tablet then follow the instructions on the screen to finish signing in. For better viewing, transfer the video to a computer or laptop. The **Samadi Yoga** site can serve as a bonus yoga library for helpful information, including a variety of articles, additional yoga classes, and a range of workshops.

You will have access to four sequences designed for each 3-month period. Please move at your own pace by starting with 20 minutes and working your way toward a 40-minute practice. You may also repeat a sequence that is more suitable for your body's level of condition.

Sequences are generally split between 20 minutes of standing or warm up postures and 20 minutes of floor postures. You may also choose to practice in 20-minute increments — practicing the standing sequence one day then practicing the floor sequence on another.

Mandalas

At the beginning of each chapter, you will discover a beautiful new mandala **to color**. This will help *reduce stress and anxiety levels and* improve your *focus and creativity.* Coloring helps with anxiety levels by relaxing the fear center of the brain — the amygdala. This induces the same state as a meditation practice, allowing the mind to momentarily release the cyclical thinking patterns. This process generates quietness and mindfulness.

Further, this "childhood" activity improves motor skills and vision, requiring the two hemispheres of the brain to communicate. Staying inside the lines uses logic, and choosing colors helps generate the creative thought process. Coloring also improves focus and concentration by activating the frontal lobe, which controls organizing and problem solving. This allows you to set everything aside and focus on the present moment. This is a great way to set yourself up for a meditation practice!

Sequence 1
40-Minute Beginner

STANDING POSES

1. **Standing Deep Breathing:** Begin with feet together or slightly apart.
   - Interlace the fingers with palms together and place hands under the chin.
   - Simultaneously inhale by the nose through 5 counts, while lifting the elbows as high as possible.
   - Hold for 1 count.
   - Exhale by the mouth for 5 counts, gently tilting the head back while bringing elbows forward and together.
   - Repeat for a total of 8 Breaths.

2. **Lunge:** Standing with feet together, place hands on hips.
   - Take a step big step forward on the right foot and slowly bend the right knee.
   - Keep the back leg straight and the back heel on the floor.
   - Be sure the right foot is directly ahead of the right hip.
   - Hold for 3 Breaths. Repeat on the left side.

3. **Standing Half Moon Pose:** Begin standing with feet together or slightly apart.
   - Inhale and reach the arms up overhead.
   - Bring the palms together and cross the thumbs.
   - Inhale and extend the upper body to the right.
   - Maintain equal weight in the feet and keep the legs and arms in straight positions.
   - Keep the chest open.
   - Hold for 3 breaths. Repeat on the other side.

4. Chair Pose: Begin standing with feet hip-width distance.
- Inhale and reach the arms forward with palms facing down and arms straight.
- Exhale and bring the hips down until the hips are slightly above the knees.
- Hold for 3 Breaths.

5. Eagle Pose: Begin with feet together and arms by the sides.
- Inhale and reach the arms up overhead.
- Exhale and bring the right arm under the left arm and wrap them around each other 1–2 times. Ideally, bring the palms together.
- Bend the knees and bring the hips down and lift the right leg over the left leg and wrap the legs around 1–2 times. If possible, wrap the toes around the back of the ankle.
- Hold the compression for 3 breaths and repeat on the left side.

6. Standing Head-to-knee, Part I: Begin standing with feet together.
- Interlace the fingers. Lift the right knee up in front and round the spine to hold the right foot in the hands. Hold the foot slightly ahead of the arch.
- Keep the standing leg straight with the left thigh muscle contracted so that the left knee is fully extended.
- Hold for 3 Breaths. Repeat on the left side.

7. Standing Bow, Part I: Begin standing with feet together.
- Bend the right knee back, lifting the foot up behind the body.
- Hold the right foot from behind. Ideally, the palm is facing outward without twisting the wrist.
- Extend the left arm straight up towards the ceiling and hold for 3 breaths. Repeat on the left side.

8. **Balancing Stick:** Begin standing with the feet together.
   - Inhale the arms straight up overhead and bring the palms together and cross the thumbs.
   - Step forward on the right foot and bring the upper body down and the left leg straight up behind you. Ideally, the upper body and left leg are parallel to the floor.
   - Hold for 3 Breaths and repeat on the left side.

9. **Separate Leg Stretching:**
   - Take a wide 4–5 foot step to the side and position the feet so they are parallel to each other.
   - Place hands on the hips and bend forward at the hips until the hands touch the floor. Straighten both legs so the knees are fully extended and the thighs are contracted.
   - Hold for 3 Breaths.

FLOOR POSES

1. **Wind Removing Pose:** Begin in a reclined position.
   - Bend the right knee and hold below the knee with fingers interlaced.
   - Pull the knee towards the shoulder and hold for 3 Breaths. Repeat on the Left side.
   - Bend both knees up and keep the knees together.
   - Reach for the opposite elbows and pull both knees in while pressing the hips down towards the floor. Try to create an extended spine against the floor. Hold for 3 breaths.

2. **Cobra Pose:** Begin lying on the stomach.
   - Place the palms underneath the chest with the fingertips in line with the top of the shoulders and the outer edge of the hands in line with the outer edges of the shoulders. Keep the legs straight and together with the tops of the feet against the floor.
   - Inhale and lift the upper body until the elbows create a 90-degree angle.
   - Hold for 3 breaths.

3. **Full Locust Pose:** Begin lying on the stomach.
   - Keep the legs together and active and reach the arms straight out to the sides with the palms downward.
   - Contract all the muscles, including the gluteus, legs, and arms. At the same time, lift the upper body, arms, and legs off the floor.
   - Hold for 3 breaths.

4. **Child's Pose:** Begin in Tabletop Position.
   - Bring the big toes together and open the knees.
   - Press the hips back towards the heels and reach the arms forward. Ideally rest the forehead on the floor.
   - Hold for 3–5 Breaths.

5. **Half Tortoise:** Sit with the hips on the heels.
   - Inhale and extend the arms overhead with the palms together.
   - Keep the arms and spine straight, and slowly hinge forward at the hips.
   - Gently place the forehead on the floor and actively reach the arms forward.
   - Keep the palms flat and pressing together, elbows extended, and simultaneously press the hips back towards the heels.
   - Hold for 3–5 Breaths

6. Camel Pose: Kneel up on the knees and place the hands on the back of the hips (glutes).
  - Lift the chest and slowly move into a backbend.
  - Carefully work to grab the heels with the hands.
  - Maintain position of the hips directly over the knees.
  - Hold for 3 breaths.
  - Place hands on hips and gently exit the pose. Sit with hips on heels, bring palms together and recover with 2–3 breaths.

7. Stretching:

Extended Leg: From a seated position.
  - Extend the right leg out at an angle and bend the left leg, placing the sole of the foot against the inner thigh.
  - Bend the right leg to grab the right foot with both hands and connect the forehead to the knee.
  - Slowly straighten the right leg while maintaining forehead-to-knee connection.
  - Keep the spine rounded. Bend the elbows down on either side of the calf.
  - Hold for 3 breaths and repeat with the left leg.

Straddle: From a seated position.
  - Spread the legs, extending both legs out at an angle and keeping the heels in the same line.
  - Walk the hands forward while keeping the legs straight. Work towards maintaining a straight spine.

Hands to Feet: Bring the legs and feet together.
  - Grab the big toes with the index and middle fingers. Work towards straightening the legs and the spine.
  - Hold for 3 to 5 breaths.

8. **Seated Extended Leg Spine Twist:** Begin with both legs out in front.
   - Bend the right knee and place the right foot outside the left knee.
   - Place the right hand behind you at the base of the spine.
   - Reach the left arm up and place the left elbow outside the right knee.
   - Inhale and lengthen the spine and exhale, twisting the spine from the lower back upward turning the neck and head last.
   - Hold for 3 breaths. Repeat on the left side.

9. **Kapalabhati Breathing (slow):** Seated comfortably with a straight spine.
   - Completely relax the abdominal muscles.
   - Visualize blowing out candles through pursed lips. Exhale and blow the "imaginary candles" out repeatedly for 40 counts. Contract the belly quickly on the exhale. If you are doing this correctly, the belly contracts back in order to force the breath out. Avoid focusing on the inhale.

1
Introduction

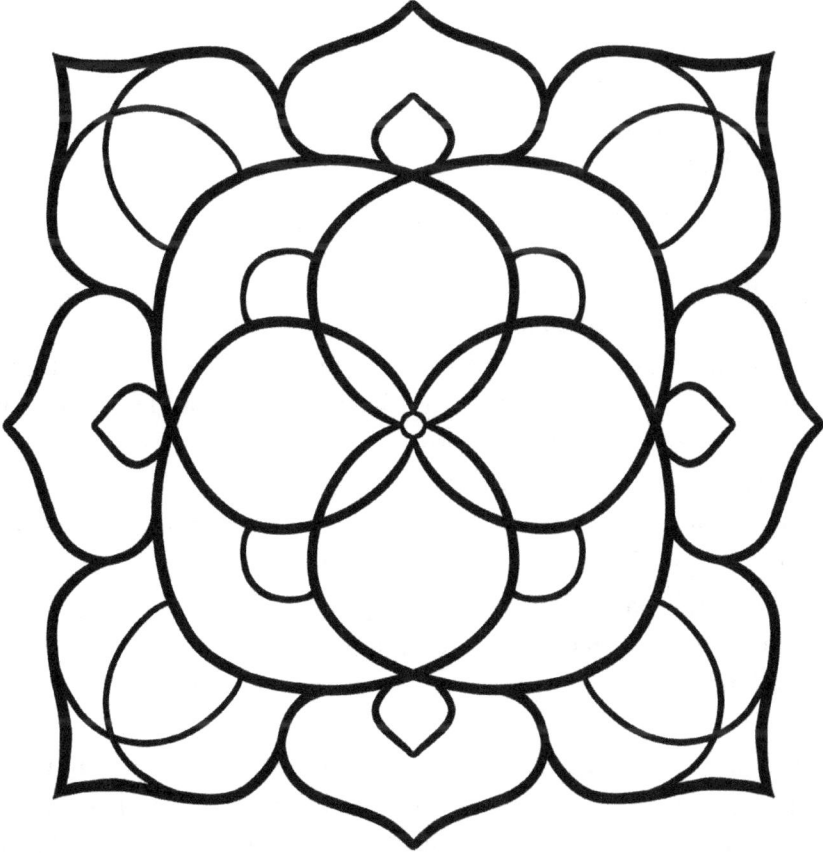

Find Your Dharma

"Instead of asking 'What do I want from life?',
a more powerful question is 'What does life want from me?'"

— *Eckhart Tolle*

In this opening chapter, I would like you to reflect on the things you enjoy in life and activities that help you feel alive. The things we enjoy *doing* are usually things we want to incorporate more in our daily life. A life well-lived fulfills a wish that makes you feel most alive and connected. It is important to find out *what* your deepest wishes or desires are to help find your Dharma. Finding your Dharma is the same as "Finding your Truth." Take a moment to reflect on what is true for you and what makes you feel alive.

The Sanskrit word Dharma comes from the root "dhri", which means to uplift or uphold. Dharma literally refers to "that which upholds righteousness and/or integrity." A sense of integrity, of purpose and inspiration, is significant on the spiritual path. To find out what is true for you, you may simply consider the following: What is important for you? What makes you feel good? What helps bring you into the present moment and in-tune with the deeper self, or in-tune with divinity? All these are questions that help you find your Dharma. A life of truth, integrity, purpose, and right action.

To find out your truth or Dharma, identify what brings you peace and joy. When we are doing something that brings us joy, we tend to be in an aware space and a present state. A joyful place is usually a more conscious space. The conscious space is where we are connected, non-judgmental, loving, and free of egoic tendencies. Conscious action includes aware actions within our-self and with the people around us. By having strong foundational yoga and meditation practices, we decrease the noise in our heads and recognize our purpose. We may discover why we were placed on this Planet. We may discover what it is that the Universe wants from us.

Realizing one's purpose does not have to be on a large scale. It also is not something that can be found somewhere in the future. To find your purpose, pay attention to moments in life that have your full attention, moments that inspire you, and possibly inspire the people around you. Most often it's in our daily living that we recognize such actions or services that bring us joy and inspire creativity.

We do not necessarily need to be in direct service to humanity; it may be in an indirect way such as creating beautiful art or music.

There is no need to search for it. Sometimes it's not even an "it", but this purpose is revealed when you are being present and aware. Most often knowing one's purpose is as simple as knowing instinctively what the next necessary step must be. If we practice patience and allow for life to unfold organically, we can tune into the messages and guidance of the Universe. This guidance only happens in the present moment when our minds are free of distractions.

Many people find purpose in activities that feel "effortless" and in some way affect their surroundings, including people or living things they serve in a positive way. The purpose that serves others, serves us simultaneously. We feel present, light, creative, connected, peaceful, and in the "flow." Pay attention to the messages from the Universe and the messages in your body, and you will know what Life wants from you.

FIND YOUR DHARMA: SELF-REFLECTION

Self-reflection Journaling 1

Part 1: Why is it important for you to have a purpose?

Part 2: What is your Dharma, Purpose, or Truth, at this moment in your life?

Part 3: How do you feel a sense of joy and fulfillment in this work?

Part 4: How will this benefit you and the community you serve?

_____

_____

_____

_____

_____

_____

_____

_____

_____

Self-reflection Journaling 2

Keep in mind that your dharma does not need to be somewhere in the future. If you can be present, you will know **what** you need to do in the next moment. Take it moment-by-moment from a space of **presence** and **awareness**. Our purpose can change and shift.

Today, what do you feel resonates most powerfully?

_____

_____

_____

_____

_____

_____

_____

_____

Self-reflection Journaling 3

When there is a lack of connection to Dharma and purpose, take a moment to be still and to be quiet. Meditate and ask the Universe to guide you.

The message does not come from outside noise, but from a deeper place.

If Dharma and purpose are not clear, **write down** the activities you enjoy.

Part 1: How do you feel **while** doing this activity? How do you feel in your physical body, emotionally and mentally?

Part 2: How do you feel **afterwards**?

Part 3: What is it about this activity that helps you feel most alive?

_____

_____

_____

_____

_____

_____

_____

_____

_____

_____

Reflect on the mental quality when you do things you enjoy. Notice how the activity takes you away from the thinking mind and helps connect you to the present moment.

Yoga and meditation will be enjoyed more fully once we become accustomed to quieting the external noise. Once the external noise is turned down, the fluctuations of the mind decrease and listening from deeper within is made possible. Some days you may consider a walk in nature as your daily meditation. During the activity, keep the mind clear, avoid labeling things such as a species of a bird or tree. Be an observer of sights, sounds, and smells. After clearing your mind, you may find an answer, or you may simply create more space and quiet for the answer to be revealed.

Yoga is for everyone, no matter the age, gender, height, weight, or background. Yoga practices are meant for *every human* to experience life fully by tuning in and unifying the health of mind, body, and soul.

COMMON MYTHS

Self-reflection Journaling 1

What are your *beliefs* or ideas about yoga, including the *types* of people who practice it?

_____

_____

_____

_____

_____

_____

_____

_____

Self-reflection Journaling 2

Part 1: What is your experience upon trying yoga and meditation?

Part 2: How does your body feel after you complete your practice? For Example, areas of tension, energy level, and overall strength?

Part 3: How do you feel emotionally after you complete your practice?

Part 4: Explain how your body may feel more energized at the end of a practice.

Part 5: How does your nervous system respond? Do you feel calmer yet energized?

Make note of how the mind fluctuates and shifts within each practice session.

Self-reflection Journaling 3

Part 1: Are you practicing at least 3 times per week? If not, what is holding you back?

Part 2: What do you notice about yourself mentally and physically when you commit to self-care and healing?

_____

_____

_____

_____

_____

_____

_____

_____

_____

_____

Self-reflection Journaling 4

Reflect on your experience of yoga practice. Do you experience a space where you are able to reconnect to your purpose? Do you have more clarity on your next necessary steps? Are you being patient and allowing messages from within to guide you towards your Purpose, Dharma, Truth?

_____

_____

_____

_____

_____

_____

_____

_____

_____

_____

_____

_____

_____

_____

_____

_____

MONTH 1 WELLNESS CALENDAR

1. On your schedule, write down each day you will practice physical yoga under the "Asana" column.

   Schedule 1 Hatha Yoga Practice each day as follows:
   Weeks 1–4: Practice 3 days per week, 20 minutes per session.

2. Write down each day you will meditate under the "Meditation" column.

   Start with 3 days per week with a 1-minute session and increase it up to 2 and 3 minutes per session.

Wellness Calendar

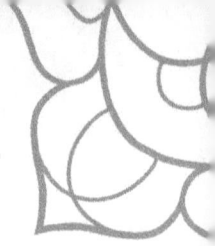

DAY	NIYAMA	ASANA	MEDITATIO
Sunday			
Monday			
Tuesday			
Wednesday			
Thursday			
Friday			
Saturday			

Month 1 _____, Week 1

OBSERVATIONS

Wellness Calendar

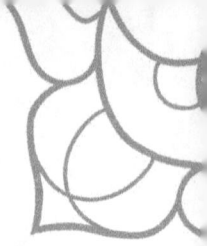

DAY	NIYAMA	ASANA	MEDITATIO
Sunday			
Monday			
Tuesday			
Wednesday			
Thursday			
Friday			
Saturday			

Month 1 _____, Week 2

OBSERVATIONS

Wellness Calendar

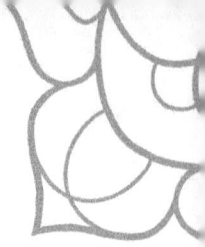

DAY	NIYAMA	ASANA	MEDITATIO
Sunday			
Monday			
Tuesday			
Wednesday			
Thursday			
Friday			
Saturday			

Month 1 _____, Week 3

OBSERVATIONS

Wellness Calendar

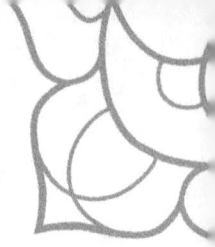

DAY	NIYAMA	ASANA	MEDITATIC
Sunday			
Monday			
Tuesday			
Wednesday			
Thursday			
Friday			
Saturday			

Month 1 _____, Week 4

OBSERVATIONS

Wellness Calendar

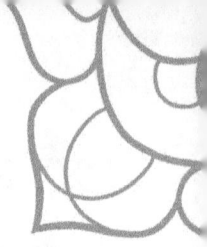

DAY	NIYAMA	ASANA	MEDITATI
Sunday			
Monday			
Tuesday			
Wednesday			
Thursday			
Friday			
Saturday			

Month 1 _____, Week 5

OBSERVATIONS

2
Finding Home

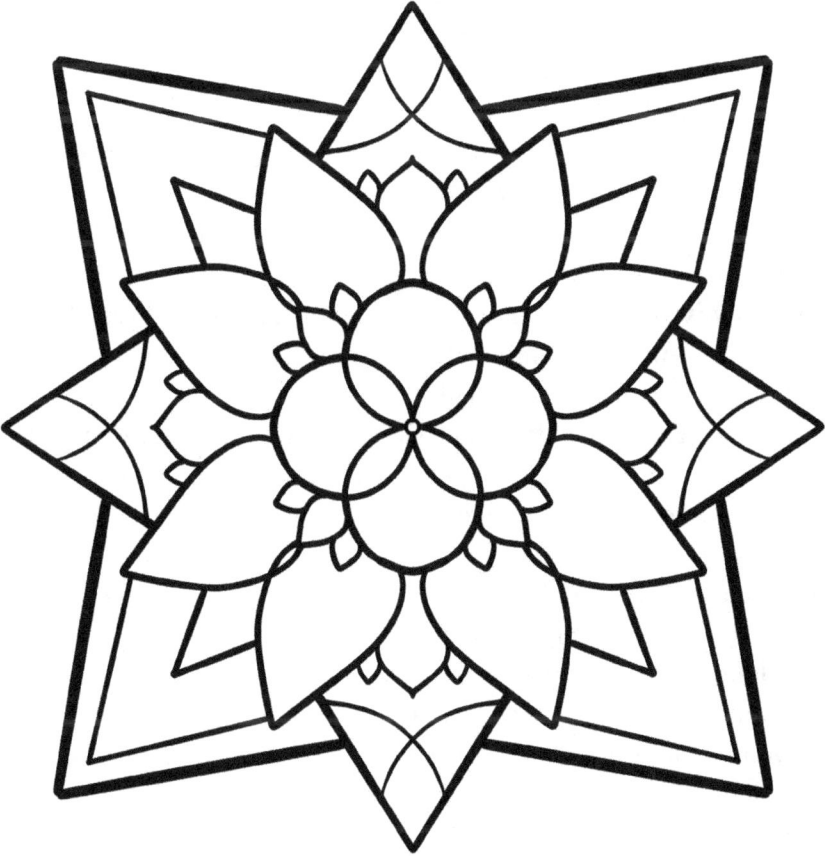

A Place or a Feeling

"Do you make regular visits to yourself?"

— *Rumi*

The concept of home begins in our formative years and usually represents an actual location. When we reflect on a childhood home, most likely we have a visual, then we may "feel" what that home was like. The feeling may resemble warmth and safety, or it may bring up anxiety and uncertainty. Luckily, as we move into adulthood, we have the ability to create a home where we feel safe, cared for, and nurtured. As we create our new home, the more important aspect is what's happening inside.

In this chapter, I would like you to discover the effects of yoga and meditation practice, and to use the practice to make regular visits to the home within. The most important home is the home inside ourselves and within our bodies. Our home within our mind and body is as — if not more — important than the physical home we live in. The more comfortable our internal home, the more comfortable the physical home will be.

A benefit of meditation and yoga practice is the calming effect to the nervous system through breath and movement. The nervous system is one that is sensitive to our mental fluctuations. Although our physical home may be safe, our internal home within mind and body may be "unsafe." The unsafe environment within is a result of our ability to handle life challenges. Most of us live free from physical danger, yet once we encounter challenges, the nervous system responds the same way as it would to a dangerous situation. The nervous system does not have the ability to differentiate between a physical danger such as a wild animal or a mental danger such as a fear of speaking in public. The perceived danger triggers the nervous system the same way since a particular thought or mental pattern results in the very same responses.

The benefits of a yoga and meditation practice include calming the nervous system and, in the process, decreasing tension in the body. An overactive and anxious mind results in short and shallow breathing, and triggers tension in the body while limiting blood flow. One of the highest benefits of yoga and meditation practice is that it puts a pause on the perpetual thinking mind to help reconnect to the flowing breath and to bring attention and release in the body *in the present moment.*

When we are anxious and worried, fear response is activated in the body. Although fear is a natural human instinct to protect and serve us in survival, much of the fear, when recognized, can be unnecessary and cause illness and disconnection. Until we find calm and comfort in our own minds and bodies, we will not find deep comfort in any other location. Everything in life is fleeting and temporary; events come and go, people come and go, and challenges come and go...and new ones arise. This is a simple fact. Unless we can create an internal world that helps us cope with challenges, we may never feel free.

Although yoga and meditation can be used to simply relieve the body of pain and calm the mind and nervous system, it can help guide us even deeper within. Yoga and meditation can be used as a spiritual practice. With yoga, we may soon begin to recognize the witnessing presence that is always there deep within. The witnessing presence is unchanging and calming. When questioning "Where is this deep presence within me?", just ask yourself *as the observer*, "Who is observing the observer?"

Self-reflection Journaling 1

Part 1: Does the word *home* generate a place or a feeling?

Part 2: Write down what you like about your home. Regarding the space, does it feel safe and comfortable?

Part 3: What item(s) can you adjust, add, or remove to make the space your own?

What beliefs or ideas can you adjust, add, or remove to make the space your own?

_____

_____

_____

_____

_____

_____

_____

_____

_____

_____

_____

_____

_____

_____

_____

_____

_____

_____

Self-reflection Journaling 2

Part 1: When facing challenges, how do you behave towards yourself and others? Are you impatient and dismissive or do you look for ways to resolve the challenge?

Part 2: How can yoga and meditation help guide you through your challenges?

Part 3: Do you believe the spiritual aspect of yoga can benefit you? Do you feel the presence within and what does this mean to you personally?

_____

_____

_____

_____

_____

_____

_____

_____

_____

_____

_____

_____

_____

Starting a meditation practice is much easier than you think. Staying with the practice is the hard part. In month 1, you began scheduling short meditation sittings 3 days per week and in month 2, I recommend increasing it to 5 days per week. Soon, I encourage you to increase your meditation practice to 7 days a week.

Write down the days you will meditate and use a timer. Set the timer for 3–5 minutes. I recommend scheduling your meditation first thing in the morning. The mental fluctuations tend to be less active in the morning so take full advantage of the calmer and slower mind.

Meditation
Tips and Techniques

Find a quiet and comfortable place in your home or space.

- Avoid meditating outside.
- Avoid using music or sounds or meditation applications.

Meditate on an empty stomach.

- Try to meditate first thing in the morning, before eating and before drinking your morning coffee or tea.

Avoid meditating with any stimulants or intoxicants in the body.

Meditate in a comfortably seated position.

- Avoid lying down to meditate.
- Ideally, use a meditation cushion.
- You may sit in a chair if there are injuries or limitations in the body.
- Make sure the spine is straight.
- If seated in a chair, avoid leaning back.
- Seat yourself with an aware, alert, yet relaxed posture.

Close your eyes.

Simply focus on the flow of the breath.

- You may choose to feel the breath moving through the nose or feel the movement of the abdomen.

Try to be still physically. Do not move or fidget in the body.

Meditation is a practice of resilience. Practice letting go of thoughts over and over again.

HEALTHY HABITS

Many of our daily routines, such as brushing our teeth and eating breakfast, are healthy and necessary. Yet, some of our habits stem from internal programming that not only hinder us but may likely be the root of most of our suffering.

Awareness practices include yoga and meditation. These practices train us to observe our thoughts, behaviors, and actions, while understanding the consequences we may suffer. Awareness practices help us observe ourselves both externally, with actions and behaviors, and internally, with our thoughts and emotions. These practices help us become observant of the outside world while staying aware of our internal mental and emotional worlds. Awareness practice is meditation and yoga because they reinforce attention on our thoughts and actions.

Later, we will delve a little deeper into mental habits that cause suffering, but let's begin with some simple habits we can easily adjust. These fundamental habits include proper hydration, nutrition, and sleep. Each of these not only affect our physical health, but our emotional and mental health too. Some slight adjustments may improve day-to-day functioning. This section will help you modify some basic health regimes that lay the "groundwork" for incorporating successful yoga and meditation practices.

As you review your water, nutrition, and sleep routines, keep in mind that the adjustments may have a big impact on cognitive function, mood, emotions, and overall physical energy. Each of the following modifications will create equilibrium throughout your day and give you a feeling of responsibility and power over your own health.

WATER AND HYDRATION

The human adult body is made up of *about 60 percent water and the vital organs: the* brain and heart are composed of 73 percent water. The lungs that are responsible for keeping us alive are about 83 percent water. Clearly, we need water for the brain, heart, and lungs to perform optimally. The lack of water causes improper brain function, which controls all aspects of bodily functions. When we discuss the negative impacts of dehydration, we usually focus on the *feeling* of dehydration rather than the true danger it poses to our internal systems and cognition. Be sure to drink the minimum daily ounces of water each day to facilitate proper functioning and to feel your best!

Self-reflection Journaling 1

Do you drink the recommended daily amount of water, which is **half of your body weight in ounces?** If yes, incorporate the recommendations on the following page, if you haven't already, and make note of improvements.

If no, then what is holding you back from addressing proper hydration?

_____

_____

_____

_____

_____

_____

_____

_____

_____

For improved hydration habits, try the following:

1. Start your day with an 8-ounce glass of room temperature water.
2. Always keep a water bottle nearby so it's accessible throughout the day.
3. Before each meal have an 8-ounce glass of water.

Self-reflection Journaling 2

Part 1: How do you feel on the days you don't drink enough water?

Part 2: How do you feel on the days you drink enough water?

Part 3: Do you tend to eat more or less when you drink enough water?

Part 4: Do you notice a difference in your energy and mood?

Part 5: Do you notice improved digestive health with proper hydration?

NUTRITION AND FOOD

Self-reflection Journaling 3

Is your daily diet a balance of proteins, fresh vegetables, and fresh fruit? How do you feel when you eat fresh fruits and vegetables in your daily diet?

Write down how you plan to incorporate more fresh and seasonal foods into your daily menu.

SLEEP

Self-reflection Journaling 4

Part 1: How many hours of sleep are you getting each night?

If it's not at least 8 hours, determine how many more hours are needed and set your new bedtime or wake-up hour.

Part 2: How do you feel when you get enough rest? How is your mood and emotional health?

Part 3: How do your habits suffer from lack of sleep? How does nutrition suffer? What happens with varying levels of caffeine and sugar consumption?

EMOTIONAL AND MENTAL HABITS

Much of our suffering and unhappiness is centered around mental habits and beliefs about ourselves. Some of these mental habits are around self-worth regarding how we evaluate and judge ourselves as a person. These beliefs are introduced to us at an early age and tend to be reinforced throughout our lives.

A toxic underlying message throughout global social systems has been in equaling a human's "worth" to the amount of wealth accumulated. Unfortunately, this belief system is not only false but extremely toxic. To evaluate our beliefs about self-worth, it is important to let go of lies and limiting ideas. These old belief systems are stories that are not true. These stories may be perpetuated through media, social media, advertising, and even pop culture. Much of the world falsely believes that self-worth is connected to net worth. This belief system keeps us detached from the deeper self and stuck in a one-dimensional perspective of the world. A limited story or belief system is usually what disconnects us, and we become stuck in unhappy places both mentally and emotionally.

If we lose our internal connection with self, we become easier targets to manipulate. If there is low self-worth or the belief that there is something lacking, then it's easier to cling to an idea or material possession to fill that void. When we feel empowered and connected within ourselves, it becomes more challenging for anyone or any belief system to have power over us.

Self-reflection Journaling 1

What is your overall self-worth based on? Is it based on your past, your family, career, or your bank account?

_____

_____

_____

_____

_____

_____

_____

_____

_____

_____

_____

_____

_____

Self-reflection Journaling 2

Do you feel you need other people to help validate who you are and your self-worth? If so, how and why?

_____

_____

_____

_____

_____

_____

_____
_____
_____
_____
_____
_____
_____
_____

Self-reflection Journaling 3

Part 1: How often do you find yourself comparing to or competing with others?

Does this make you feel more valuable or less valuable?

Part 2: Reflect on your emotional state. How does comparing yourself to others make you feel? How does comparing your life to other people's lives make you feel?

Do you believe that your self-worth is based on a "winning or losing" storyline?

What are the feelings and/or sensations in your body when you compare yourself to others?

_____
_____
_____
_____

_____

_____

_____

_____

_____

_____

_____

_____

_____

_____

_____

_____

_____

_____

_____

Self-reflection Journaling 4

It is important to learn to nurture and love ourselves.

Practice telling yourself each day, "I love you." If this is too challenging, then tell yourself "I see you." The goal is to focus the attention inward and create a safe and loving space from within.

Part 1: How often do you tell yourself *you love you* or *you see you*?

Part 2: Is this comfortable or uncomfortable to do and if so, why?

Part 3: What feelings does this experience of *self-nurturing* bring up for you?

_____

_____

_____

_____

_____

_____

_____

_____

_____

_____

_____

_____

_____

_____

_____

Recognize that the deeper self is the *witnessing presence*. The deeper self or true self does not change based on your age, finances, your career, what you achieve, or don't achieve. It is not dependent on your name, belief system or any concept. This deeper self is consciousness and beyond anything one can conceptually name or describe. Remind yourself of this the next time you question your worth.

ELIMINATE THE NOISE

Technology today is designed to attract you and distract you at the same time. Technology is a huge market competing to get the most attention and the biggest profits. Social Media, Streaming Services, Applications, and even your email's mailbox design are engineered to grab your attention. It is very important to notice how many times you check your phone, messages, emails, and social media. Instead of getting trapped "by design", make it a habit to create some space from all advertising, media, and technology.

Try to take a day, half-a-day, or several hours each week to detach from smartphones, smartwatches, laptops, and other devices. Take time to turn off all external distractions. Experience the freedom you create by temporarily eliminating the external noise. Recognize that the noise is keeping you from feeling and connecting to yourself.

Self-reflection Journaling 1

How many of your daily hours are consumed by smartphones, laptops, and devices?

Do you notice that you become obsessed and affected by what you see or read? How?

Self-reflection Journaling 2

How do you feel physically, mentally, and emotionally when consuming advertising, news stories, or social media?

Do you believe this benefits you in any way? How?

_____

_____

_____

_____

_____

_____

_____

MONTH 2 WELLNESS CALENDAR

On your schedule, write down each day you will practice.

Schedule Hatha Yoga Practice as follows:
Weeks 1–4: Practice 3 times per week. At least one day/week practice for 40-min.

Schedule Meditation Practice as follows:
3 days per week, using a timer

Week 1: Morning Only: 5 minutes each day

Week 2: Morning Only: 10 minutes each day

Week 3: 10-minute morning meditation _and_
       5-minute evening meditation

Week 4: 10-minute morning meditation _and_
       10-minute evening meditation

Wellness Calendar

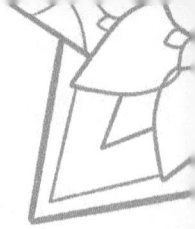

DAY	NIYAMA	ASANA	MEDITATIO
Sunday			
Monday			
Tuesday			
Wednesday			
Thursday			
Friday			
Saturday			

Month 2 _____, Week 1

OBSERVATIONS

Wellness Calendar

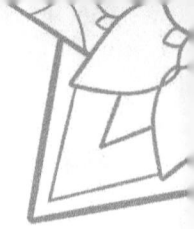

DAY	NIYAMA	ASANA	MEDITATIC
Sunday			
Monday			
Tuesday			
Wednesday			
Thursday			
Friday			
Saturday			

Month 2 _____, Week 2

OBSERVATIONS

Wellness Calendar

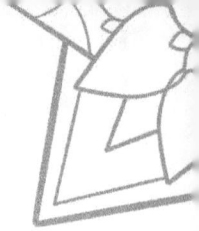

DAY	NIYAMA	ASANA	MEDITATI
Sunday			
Monday			
Tuesday			
Wednesday			
Thursday			
Friday			
Saturday			

Month 2 _____, Week 3

OBSERVATIONS

Wellness Calendar

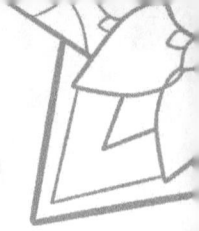

DAY	NIYAMA	ASANA	MEDITATIO
Sunday			
Monday			
Tuesday			
Wednesday			
Thursday			
Friday			
Saturday			

Month 2 _____, Week 4

OBSERVATIONS

Wellness Calendar

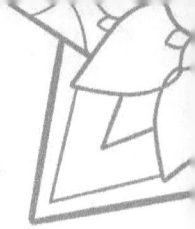

DAY	NIYAMA	ASANA	MEDITATIO
Sunday			
Monday			
Tuesday			
Wednesday			
Thursday			
Friday			
Saturday			

Month 2 _____, Week 5

OBSERVATIONS

3

Samadhi

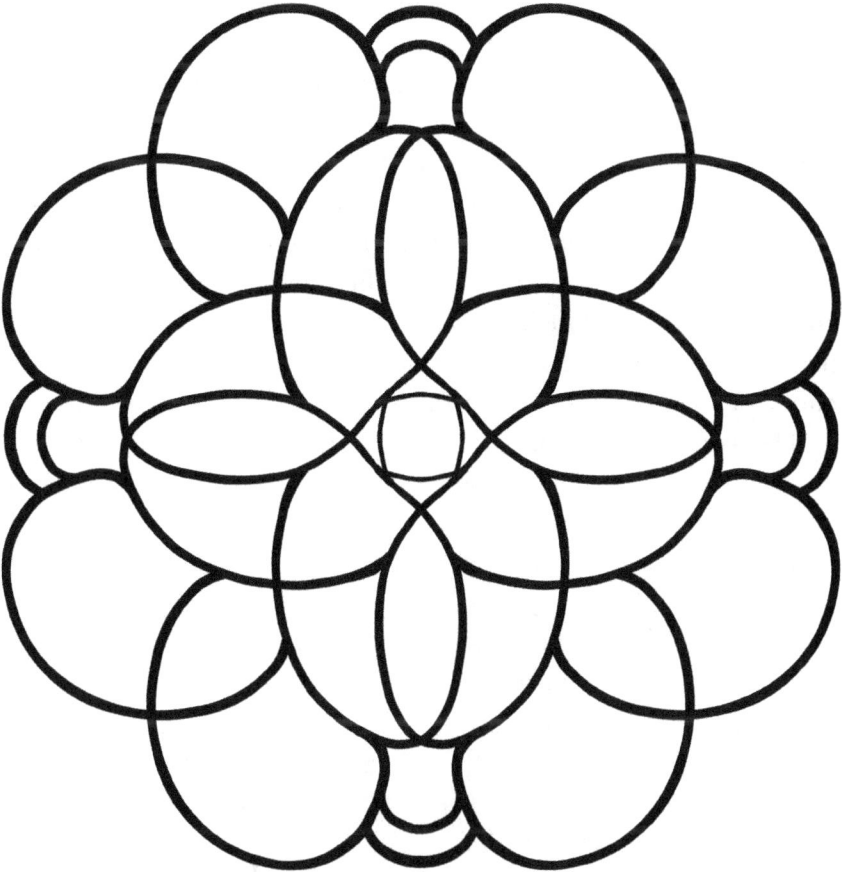

The 8th Limb of Yoga

"The primary cause of unhappiness is never the situation
but your thoughts about it."

— *Eckhart Tolle*

My journey to self-healing started when I began my practice of Meditation and Yoga. I turned to yoga to find a way to suffer less mentally, emotionally, and physically. The beauty of yoga and meditation is that the healing happens within one's own experience of the practices. Samadhi, meaning mastery of the mind, is the eighth limb of Patanjali's Yoga Sutras and the final stage of self-realization. The sutras teach us different facets of how to embody yoga in mind, body, and spirit. Patanjali was believed to be a sage who was one of the first to arrange yoga philosophy in a written format around 1,700 years ago.

In this Chapter, I would like you to discover how using yoga and meditation practices can and will improve the many dimensions of your life. These dimensions include the physical, mental, emotional and spiritual layers. Much of our suffering begins in our mind and is magnified by how we handle challenges. Some basic yoga philosophy and yoga practice can help us with less suffering and more peace.

The preceding 7 limbs of yoga put us on a path of right and conscious action. Conscious action means we are aware of internal and external feedback within ourselves. We conduct ourselves with awareness so as to avoid being governed by stories or belief systems. With conscious actions, we avoid judgement mentality which creates isolation within ourselves and towards others. As humans, we are not designed to be solitary; we are inter-connected at the root of our being. The 8 limbs of yoga lead us toward a life of compassion for both ourselves and others, with awareness, love, and care. With these disciplines and "right actions," we reduce conflicts and dramas in daily life, resulting in less suffering.

Much of our anguish is magnified by overthinking and obsessing over events that either have or have not happened. This is considered past and future thinking. We may even cling to past stories or belief systems that no longer serve us or benefit our relationships. Much of this suffering is magnified by a hyper-active and fluctuating mind that is unobserved.

The practice of yoga and meditation puts a "pause" on incessant thinking, reconnects us to the body, breath, and the present moment, and allows for a deeper connection to the self. The body and the breath *bring our attention back* to the present moment while the thinking mind *takes us out* of the present moment. When we are lost in perpetual thinking, we are apt to be in a constant state of worry, doubt, and fear. These are negative tendencies that disconnect us from reality and keep us stuck in unhappy cycles.

Life is constantly challenging us. This fact is something to accept, not fear. Growth comes from challenges. They lead us to wisdom and build our resiliency. The white lotus flower is a wonderful representation of awakening and an accurate symbol of our life process. From "challenging" unclear and muddy waters, the lotus flower emerges into full beauty, life, consciousness. To handle these tests, we are best served by reinforcing our emotional, mental, and physical health. Mastery of the mind — Samadhi — takes practice, discipline, and self-reflection.

Meditation and mindfulness practices reduce activity in the amygdala, an area of the brain that governs the fight or flight stress response as well as fear and emotion. Researchers have observed human brains, with the use of brain scans, that reveal just 10 continuous sessions of meditation help to not only reduce the reactivity in the amygdala during upsetting situations, but also to recover more quickly after a stressful event occurs.

To conclude, meditation is a proven tool for resilience and mental health.

MONTH 3 WELLNESS CALENDAR

On your schedule, write down each day you will practice.
Schedule Hatha Yoga practice as follows:
Weeks 1–4: Practice 3 days per week. At least 2 days a week, practice for 40-minutes

Schedule Meditation Practice as follows:
5 days per week, using a timer
Week 1: Morning only, 5 minutes each day.
Week 2: Morning only, 10 minutes each day
Week 3: 10-minute morning and 5-minute evening meditation
Week 4: 10-minute morning and 10-minute evening meditation

Wellness Calendar

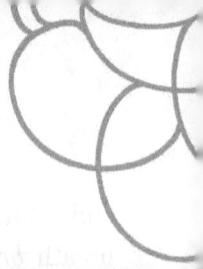

DAY	NIYAMA	ASANA	MEDITATIO
Sunday			
Monday			
Tuesday			
Wednesday			
Thursday			
Friday			
Saturday			

Month 3 _____, Week 1

OBSERVATIONS

Wellness Calendar

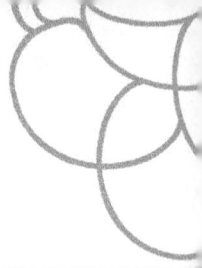

DAY	NIYAMA	ASANA	MEDITATI
Sunday			
Monday			
Tuesday			
Wednesday			
Thursday			
Friday			
Saturday			

Month 3 _____, Week 2

OBSERVATIONS

Wellness Calendar

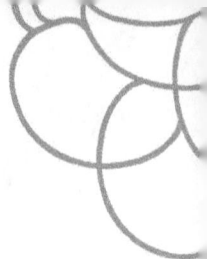

DAY	NIYAMA	ASANA	MEDITATIC
Sunday			
Monday			
Tuesday			
Wednesday			
Thursday			
Friday			
Saturday			

Month 3 _____, Week 3

OBSERVATIONS

Wellness Calendar

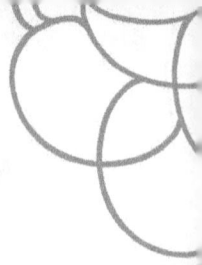

DAY	NIYAMA	ASANA	MEDITATI
Sunday			
Monday			
Tuesday			
Wednesday			
Thursday			
Friday			
Saturday			

Month 3 _____, Week 4

OBSERVATIONS

Wellness Calendar

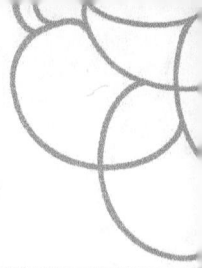

DAY	NIYAMA	ASANA	MEDITATIO
Sunday			
Monday			
Tuesday			
Wednesday			
Thursday			
Friday			
Saturday			

Month 3 _____, Week 5

OBSERVATIONS

Sequence 2
40-Minute Beginner/Intermediate

STANDING POSES

1. **Standing Pranayama Deep Breathing:** Begin with feet together or slightly apart.
   - Interlace the fingers with palms together and place hands under the chin.
   - Simultaneously inhale by the nose through 6 counts, while lifting the elbows as high as possible.
   - Hold for 1 count.
   - Exhale by the mouth for 6 counts, gently tilting the head back while bringing elbows forward and together.
   - Repeat for a total of 8 Breaths.

2. **Lunge (with back heel over toes):** Begin standing with feet together, place hands on hips.
   - Take a step big step forward on the right foot and slowly bend the right knee.
   - Keep the back leg straight and lift the back heel until the heel is directly over the toes.
   - Be sure the right foot is directly ahead of the right hip.
   - Inhale arms overhead and bring the palms together.
   - Hold for 3 Breaths. Repeat on the left side.

3. Standing Half Moon Pose with Backbend and Hands to Feet Pose

Half Moon: Begin standing with feet together or slightly apart.
- Inhale and reach the arms up overhead.
- Bring the palms together and cross the thumbs.
- Inhale and extend the upper body to the right.
- Maintain equal weight in the feet and keep the legs and arms in straight positions.
- Keep the chest open.
- Hold for 3 breaths. Repeat on the other side.

Backbend: Keep arms extended straight up and engage the gluteus muscles.
- Lift the chest and slowly move into a backbend. Find the depth where you can maintain the position and hold for 3 breaths.

Forward Bend to Hands to Feet Pose
- Slowly move into a forward fold and grab the heels (or ankles).
- Connect the legs to the upper body and slowly straighten the legs and stretch the spine downward.
- Maintain upper and lower body connection and hold for 3 breaths.

4. Chair Pose (3 parts):

Part I: Begin standing with feet hip-width distance.
- Inhale and reach the arms forward with palms facing down and arms straight.
- Exhale and bring the hips down until the hips are slightly above the knees.
- Hold for 3 Breaths.

Part II: Keep the feet hip-width distance and arms parallel to the floor.
- Lift the heels until the heels are over the toes.
- Contract the leg, glute and abdominal muscles and slowly bend the knees, until the hips are slightly above the knees. Maintain the position of the heels directly over the toes.
- Hold for 3 breaths.

Part III, Classic Chair:
- Bring the feet and knees together.
- Lift the arms upward at an angle and sit the hips down. Keep the feet and knees together and hold for 3 breaths.

5. **Eagle Pose:** Begin with feet together and arms by the sides.
- Inhale and reach the arms up overhead.
- Exhale and bring the right arm under the left arm and wrap them around each other 1–2 times. Ideally, bring the palms together.
- Bend the knees and bring the hips down and lift the right leg over the left leg and wrap the legs around 1–2 times. If possible, wrap the toes around the back of the ankle.
- Hold the compression for 3 breaths and repeat on the left side.

6. **Standing Head-to-knee, Parts I & II:** Begin standing with feet together.

Part I
- Interlace the fingers. Lift the right knee up in front and round the spine to hold the right foot in the hands. Hold the foot slightly ahead of the arch.
- Keep the standing leg straight with the left thigh muscle contracted so that the left knee is fully extended.

Part II

- Slowly extend the right leg forward and until the heel is at the same level as the right hip. Keep the abdominal muscles contracted and the spine rounded. Extend the right leg until the knee is fully extended and the thigh contracted.
- Keep both knees extended and both thighs contracted and the spine rounded. Hold for 3 Breaths. Repeat on the left side.

7. **Standing Bow:** Begin standing with feet together.
   - Bend the right knee back, lifting the foot up behind the body.
   - Hold the right foot from behind. Ideally, the palm is facing outward (without twisting the wrist).
   - Extend the left arm straight up towards the ceiling.
   - Begin pressing the right foot back into the hand to create a backbend.
   - Slowly bring the torso and upper body downward toward the floor. Hold for 3 Breaths. Repeat on the left side.

8. **Balancing Stick:** Begin standing with the feet together.
   - Inhale the arms straight up overhead and bring the palms together and cross the thumbs.
   - Step forward on the right foot and bring the upper body down and the left leg straight up behind you.
   - Maintain a straight line from the fingertips to the left toes. Work towards bringing the upper body and left leg parallel to the floor.
   - Hold for 3 Breaths and repeat on the left side.

9. **Separate Leg Stretching:** Begin standing with the feet together.
   - Take a wide 4–5 foot step to the side and position the feet so they are parallel to each other. Arms are stretched outward and parallel to the floor.
   - Bend forward at the hips and grab your heels. Straighten both legs so the knees are fully extended and the thighs are contracted.
   - Gently pull with the arms and touch the forehead to the floor between the feet.
   - Hold for 3 Breaths.

10. **Triangle Pose:** Begin with the feet together.
    - Take a 5-foot step to the right, and stretch the arms to the sides so they are parallel to the floor.
    - Turn the right foot until it's parallel to the edge of the mat. Turn the left foot inward slightly.
    - Bend the right knee until the hip is at the level of the knee and the knee is directly over the right ankle. Maintain a straight left leg.
    - Move arms together and place the right elbow in front of the right knee while reaching the right arm downward. At the same time reach the left arm straight upward so that the arms together form one straight line.
    - Keep the lift hip forward slightly, bring the left shoulder back, and look up towards the palm of the left hand.
    - Hold for 3 breaths. Repeat on the left side.

11. **Separate Leg Forehead-to-knee:** Begin standing with the feet together and the arms extended straight up overhead with the palms together.
    - Take a 3-foot step to the right, and lift the toes and rotate on the heels so that the right foot is forward and the back foot is turned

at an angle. Keep the arms extended straight upward and palms together.
- Bring the chin down and slowly articulate the spine while rounding forward until the forehead touches the right knee. Bend the knee as much as needed.
- Keep arms extended forward ahead of the right foot.
- Hold for 3 breaths. Repeat on the left side.

12. **Tree Pose:** Begin standing with the feet together.
- Lift the right knee in front of the body as high as possible and gently bring the right foot to the top of the left thigh.
- Keep the standing leg straight. Contract the abdominal and gluteus muscles and stand tall. Hold for 3 breaths. Repeat on the the left side.

FLOOR POSES

1. **Wind Removing Pose :** Begin in a reclined position.
- Bend the right knee and hold below the knee with fingers interlaced.
- Pull the knee towards the shoulder so that the thigh is alongside the ribs and hold for 3 Breaths. Repeat on the Left side.
- Bend both knees up and keep the knees together.
- Reach for the opposite elbows and pull both knees in while pressing the hips down towards the floor. Try to create an extended spine against the floor. Hold for 3 breaths.

2. Cobra: Begin lying on the stomach.
- Place the palms underneath the chest with the fingertips in line with the top of the shoulders and the outer edge of the hands in line with the outer edges of the shoulders. Keep the legs straight and together with the tops of the feet against the floor.
- Inhale and lift the upper body until the elbows create a 90-degree angle.
- Hold for 3 breaths.

3. Locust: Begin lying on the stomach.
- Place the chin on the floor and bring the arms into a straight position underneath the body, pointing towards the feet. The palms should be flat on the floor and the fingers spread out.
- Inhale and lift the right leg up to 45-degrees. Keep the right hip against the right forearm. Continuously press both hands and shoulders against the floor. Hold for 3 breaths and repeat with the left leg.
- Place the mouth on the floor. Inhale, engage the gluteus and leg muscles and lift both legs together. Keep the legs together, thighs contracted and feet touching. Hold for 3 breaths.

4. Full Locust: Begin lying on the stomach.
- Keep the legs together and active and reach the arms straight out to the sides with the palms downward.
- Contract all the muscles, including the gluteus, legs, and arms. At the same time, lift the upper body, arms, and legs off the floor.
- Hold for 3 breaths.

5. Bow Pose: Begin face-down with the chin on the floor.
- Bend both legs at the knees and grab the feet from the outside, halfway between the toes and heels.

- Engage the gluteus muscles, inhale, and actively kick the legs back and up. Hold for 3 breaths.
- Bring the palms under the chest and press the body up into a **Tabletop or Quadruped position**.

6. Child's Pose: Begin in Tabletop or Quadruped Position.
- Bring the big toes together and open the knees.
- Press the hips back towards the heels and reach the arms forward, bending forward and bring the forehead to the floor.
- Hold for 3–5 Breaths.

7. Half Tortoise: Sit with the hips on the heels. Knees and feet touching.
- Inhale and extend the arms overhead with the palms together.
- Keep the arms and spine straight, and slowly hinge forward at the hips.
- Gently place the forehead on the floor and actively reach the arms forward.
- Keep the palms flat and pressing together, edge of pinky fingers touch the floor, elbows extended, and simultaneously press the hips back towards the heels.
- Hold for 3–5 Breaths

8. Camel Pose: Kneel up on the knees and place the hands on the back of the hips (glutes).
- Lift the chest and slowly move into a backbend.
- Carefully work to grab the heels with the hands.
- Maintain position of the hips directly over the knees.
- Hold for 3 Breaths.

9. This being the deepest backbend. Take a rest at this point by lying on your back in Savasana or sit with hips on heels and press palms together. Take 3–5 Breaths.

10. **Rabbit Pose:** Begin sitting on your heels with the feet together.
    - Grab the heels with the thumbs on the outside and the fingertips on the inside of the heels. Make sure you have a tight grip.
    - Contract the abdominal muscles, bring the chin down and slowly round your spine forward to bring the forehead to the knees.
    - Slowly lift the hips while simultaneously pulling on the heels. Avoid placing weight in the top of the head. Only a slight amount is safe. Keep the feet touching each other and against the floor and hold for 3 Breaths.

11. **Stretching:**
    Extended Leg Stretch: From a seated position.
    - Extend the right leg out at an angle and bend the left leg, placing the sole of the foot against the inner thigh.
    - Bend the right leg to grab the right foot with both hands and connect the forehead to the knee.
    - Slowly straighten the right leg while maintaining forehead-to-knee connection.
    - Keep the spine rounded. Bend the elbows down on either side of the calf.
    - Hold for 3 breaths and repeat with the left leg.
    Straddle Stretch: From a seated position.
    - Spread the legs, extending both legs out at an angle and keeping the heels in the same line.
    - Walk the hands forward while keeping the legs straight. Work towards maintaining a straight spine.

Hands to Feet Stretch: Bring the legs and feet together.
- Hook the big toes with the index and middle fingers.
- Try to touch the stomach to the thighs and then the chest to the knees.
- Work on straightening the legs and the spine. You may have to work on one at a time.
- Hold for 3 to 5 breaths.

12. **Spine Twist with Bent Legs:** Begin with both legs out in front.
    - Bend the right knee and place the right foot outside the left knee.
    - Bend the left knee and place the left foot outside the right hip. Make sure both sides of the hips are evenly on the floor.
    - Place the right hand behind you at the base of the spine.
    - Reach the left arm up and place the left elbow outside the right knee.
    - Inhale and lengthen the spine and exhale, twisting the spine from the lower back upward so that the head and neck turn last.
    - Hold for 3 breaths. Repeat on the left side.

13. **Kapalabhati Breathing (faster rhythm):** Begin seated comfortably with a straight spine.
    - Completely relax the abdominal muscles.
    - Visualize blowing out candles through pursed lips. Exhale and blow the imaginary candles out repeatedly for 50 counts at a fast and even pace. Contract the belly quickly on the exhale. If you are doing this correctly, the belly contracts back in order to force the breath out. Avoid focusing on the inhale.

4
Meditation

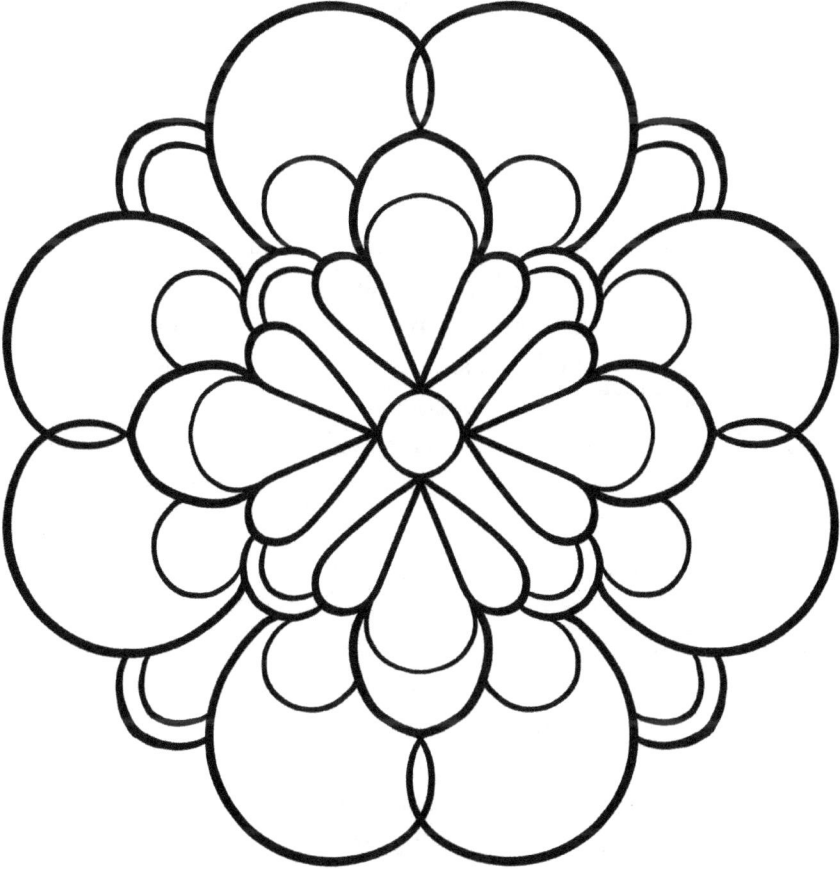

The Essential Component of Yoga

"Being must be felt. It can't be thought"

— *Eckhart Tolle*

According to Buddhist philosophy, life is full of suffering, and the way to eliminate suffering is through cessation of mental attachment and resistance.

A positive effect of the 2020 global pandemic was the many people turning to meditation to help calm the nervous system to lower anxiety levels. In addition to the calming effects, the practice of meditation improves our mental resilience and reinforces non-reactivity.

Non-reactivity doesn't mean to reduce our care, concern, or compassion in challenging events. Instead, non-reactivity results from mental training, which keeps us aware, connected to the breath, and rooted in the reality of the moment. When an upsetting event occurs, rather than attaching or resisting the event, we learn to be in the present moment. It is a simple practice that helps us stay fully aware of the NOW and less reactive to the dramas of life.

In this chapter, I would like you to focus on your meditation practices. Make them your priority each week and each day, while recognizing the positive effects. Notice how meditation starts your day by reducing anxiety, slowing the thoughts, and tuning into the breath. Meditation practice is challenging and rewarding. It only takes a couple of minutes a day to begin the discipline. Be patient and kind towards yourself but commit to sitting each morning and focusing on the breath with awareness, alertness, grace, and patience. Keep in mind you're not forcing yourself *not* to think but building the discipline of focusing on the breath. Notice the thoughts and let them go. This is a practice of resilience.

A typical meditation sitting begins with focus on the breath, a thought arises, you notice it, you let it go, then you focus back on the breath. Another thought arises, you notice it, you let it go, and focus back on the breath. Many times, the thought will hook you and you continue down the path of more thoughts. The goal is to notice and go back to the breath.... Over and over again.

Meditation is not the absence of thought; it is the active observation of thought without analysis. When we learn to observe a thought, we create space and avoid attaching to or resisting it. In addition to affecting the *amygdala*, meditation affects the *default network* of the brain.

Our brain's default mode can be described as mind-wandering. For most of us, even when we're doing nothing, our brains are highly active. Work projects, to-do lists and worrying about finances may feel like the norm but can be quite taxing on the brain. This specific area of the brain called the *default network* manages all that mind-wandering, and it requires energy and resources that are also needed for memory and cognition. Over time, the more energy and resources that go to the default network, the fewer you have available for paying attention and remembering other things.

Self-reflection Journaling 1

Do you notice a difference in yourself on days you practice meditation? How?

Do you notice results with the increased frequency of practice? How?

_____

_____

_____

_____

_____

Self-reflection Journaling 2

Do you feel your patience improved? If so, with who and what events?

Are you feeling more compassion for yourself and the people around you? How?

_____

_____

_____

_____

_____

_____

_____

_____

_____

_____

_____

Self-reflection Journaling 3

Much of our energy depletion is due to over-thinking and giving in to an over-active mind.

Do you feel clearer mentally on the days you meditate? How? If not, increase consistency and duration and then make note of the results.

Do you have more mental energy and a "higher bandwidth" on the days you meditate? If not, increase your consistency and duration and make note of the results.

_____

_____

_____

_____

_____

_____

_____

_____

_____

_____

_____

_____

_____

_____

_____

_____

_____

Self-reflection Journaling 4

Know that each day is different, and, on most days, meditation is challenging. When fluctuations are higher, try to meditate a little longer. It may take more time to find the focus.

Do you notice mental fluctuations vary from day-to-day? Do the fluctuations vary based on current life events? How do you feel with a longer meditation sitting and increased frequency of practice?

Self-reflection Journaling 5

Much of our suffering comes from *clinging to* and *replaying* certain thoughts.

Recognize that replaying certain thoughts can be a form of mental abuse towards self.

Remember you cannot "will" yourself to stop thinking, but you can practice bringing the attention back to the breath in the present moment. Once we acknowledge that thoughts are just "thoughts" which come and go like clouds in the sky, then we can learn to simply be observers of these thoughts. We learn to simply let them go. This is a practice of mental resilience.

During your meditation practice are you being kind to yourself?

Are you practicing observing the thoughts that come and go *with patience and kindness*?

Are you practicing *not attaching* to these thoughts? How?

_____

_____

_____

_____

_____

_____

_____

MONTH 4 WELLNESS CALENDAR

On your schedule, write down each day you will practice.

Schedule Hatha Yoga Practice as follows:
Weeks 1–4: Practice 3 days per week; Increase all 3 practices to 40 minutes each.

Schedule Meditation Practice as follows:
7 days per week, using a timer
Week 1–2: 10-minute morning meditation
Week 3: 10-minute morning meditation *and*
      5-minute evening meditation
Week 4: 10-minute morning meditation *and*
      10-minute evening meditation

Wellness Calendar

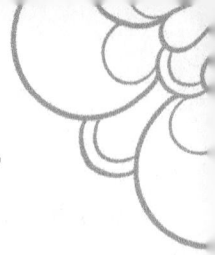

DAY	NIYAMA	ASANA	MEDITATION
Sunday			
Monday			
Tuesday			
Wednesday			
Thursday			
Friday			
Saturday			

Month 4 _____, Week 1

OBSERVATIONS

Wellness Calendar

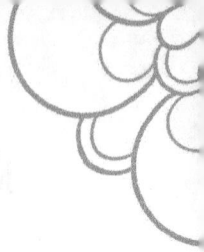

DAY	NIYAMA	ASANA	MEDITATI
Sunday			
Monday			
Tuesday			
Wednesday			
Thursday			
Friday			
Saturday			

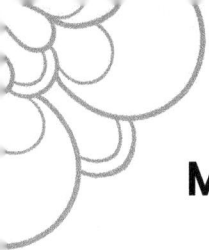

Month 4 _____, Week 2

OBSERVATIONS

Wellness Calendar

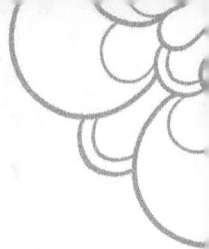

DAY	NIYAMA	ASANA	MEDITATION
Sunday			
Monday			
Tuesday			
Wednesday			
Thursday			
Friday			
Saturday			

Month 4 _____, Week 3

OBSERVATIONS

Wellness Calendar

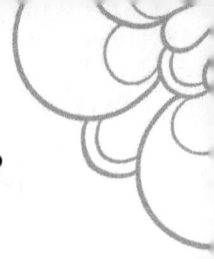

DAY	NIYAMA	ASANA	MEDITATIO
Sunday			
Monday			
Tuesday			
Wednesday			
Thursday			
Friday			
Saturday			

Month 4 _____, Week 4

OBSERVATIONS

Wellness Calendar

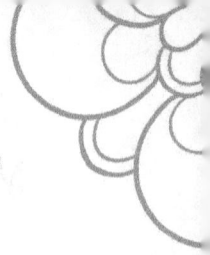

DAY	NIYAMA	ASANA	MEDITATI
Sunday			
Monday			
Tuesday			
Wednesday			
Thursday			
Friday			
Saturday			

Month 4 _____, Week 5

OBSERVATIONS

5

Hatha Yoga

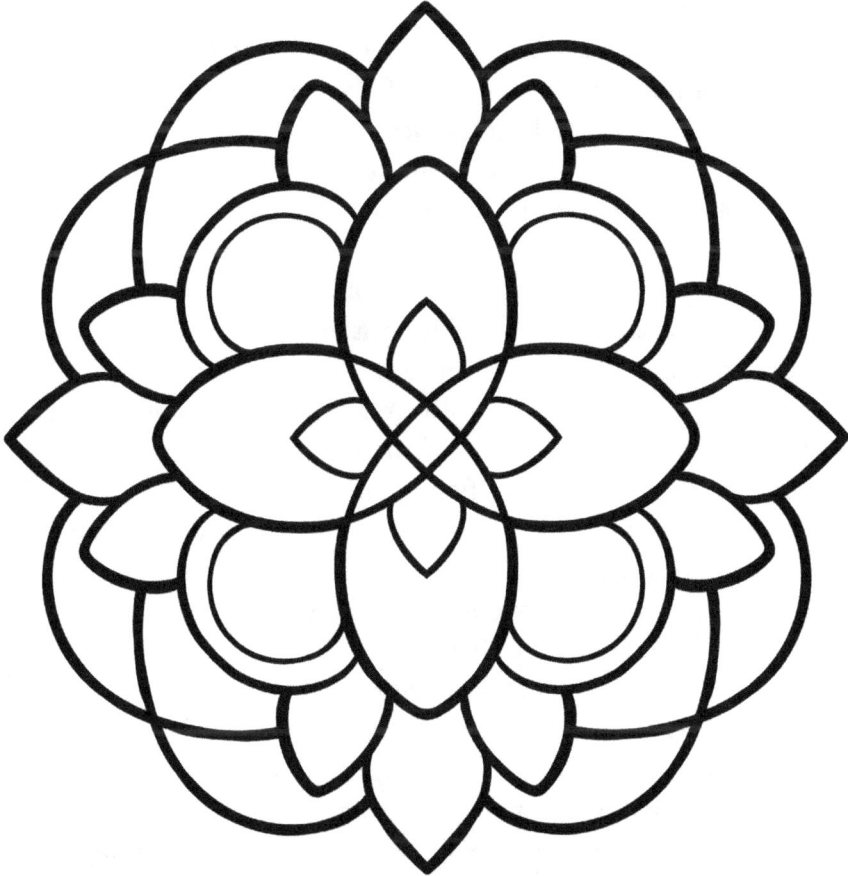

Physical Practice & Breathing Techniques

"Awareness is the greatest agent for change."

— *Eckhart Tolle*

Hatha Yoga, the most common form of yoga practiced today in the West, is a physical practice along with Pranayams, which are breathing techniques. The intention of Hatha Yoga, which blossomed about a thousand years ago, was to prepare the body for the more advanced practices of meditation and insight. The Sanskrit translation for Hatha is *fierce and forceful*. This definition refers to the physicality of the practice but is not intended to force the body brutally past its capability. Instead, the Hatha aspect of yoga takes physical effort to condition the body with strength and flexibility through regular practice, always with the intent to avoid injury and self-harm.

In this chapter, my wish for you is to increase body awareness through your physical practice and to allow the same awareness to the thinking patterns that offer insight on your actions and behaviors. This is only one part of the overall scope of yoga for unifying mind, body, and soul. Once Hatha Yoga practice is done with consistency, you create a strong foundation to move to the next steps of extended meditations and self-observations.

Hatha — pronounced Hah-dha — was developed to prepare the body to sit for long periods of time. It was acknowledged early on that most adults cannot comfortably sit on the floor in a cross-legged easy pose for any length of time.

For most people, it is much easier to move the body than to sit still and observe the mind. The discipline of physical yoga may be considered a prerequisite to sitting meditation.

A physical practice is intended to focus attention on the breath and the body. The physical practice of Hatha Yoga helps us pay attention to areas of the body and observe the information through bodily sensations. This teaches awareness practice. Tuning into the bodily sensations momentarily helps disengage from perpetual thinking.

You may practice this now: Take a moment to feel your feet on the floor. How do your feet feel at this moment? Do you feel warmth, cold, tingling or vibration? While you are in a state of awareness to sense the feeling, it is practically impossible to be stuck in another thought. This "awareness" practice helps you take a moment to step out of thinking and move into feeling. The sensations, energy and aliveness in your body are what is happening now. The thinking in your mind may have nothing to do with the **now** but most likely about something in the past or future. Hatha Yoga practice serves as a "steppingstone" to bring awareness to the body and breath which will prepare you for the more challenging seated meditation and introspection practices.

Self-Reflection Journaling 1

During Hatha Yoga practice, are you staying in touch with the breath? Do you notice the result of the pose when you hold your breath? How is the pose different when you are in touch with the flow of the breath?

Are you using your breath as an indicator to how far you can move into a pose? How?

What happens to the breath when you are pushing the body too far?

The body's way of communicating is with pain sensations. Can you differentiate "bad pain" from the sensation of building proper strength and flexibility? How?

Self-Reflection Journaling 2

Do you notice your practice varies based on your mental fluctuations?

Are you noticing habitual messaging during your practice? Judgment, dissatisfaction, comparison or competition?

When holding a pose, do you find yourself struggling to hold a pose? When you notice the struggle, are you thinking or holding your breath? What happens when you focus on the breath and learn to surrender to the pose no matter how challenging?

MONTH 5 WELLNESS CALENDAR

On your schedule, write down each day you will practice.

Schedule Hatha Yoga Practice (20–40mins each) as follows:
Week 1: Practice 3 days
Week 2: Practice 3 days
Week 3: Practice 5 days
Week 4: Practice 5 days

Schedule Meditation Practice 7 days per week as follows:
Weeks 1–4: 10-minute morning meditation

Wellness Calendar

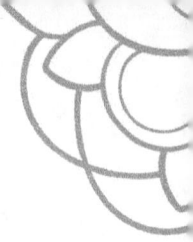

DAY	NIYAMA	ASANA	MEDITATIO
Sunday			
Monday			
Tuesday			
Wednesday			
Thursday			
Friday			
Saturday			

Month 5 _____, Week 1

OBSERVATIONS

Wellness Calendar

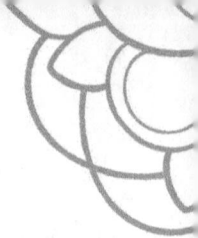

DAY	NIYAMA	ASANA	MEDITATION
Sunday			
Monday			
Tuesday			
Wednesday			
Thursday			
Friday			
Saturday			

Month 5 _____, Week 2

OBSERVATIONS

Wellness Calendar

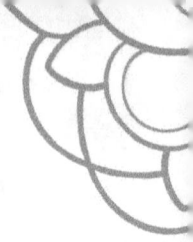

DAY	NIYAMA	ASANA	MEDITATI
Sunday			
Monday			
Tuesday			
Wednesday			
Thursday			
Friday			
Saturday			

Month 5 _____, Week 3

OBSERVATIONS

Wellness Calendar

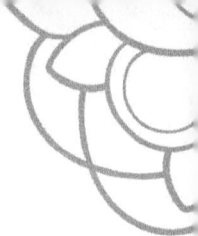

DAY	NIYAMA	ASANA	MEDITATI
Sunday			
Monday			
Tuesday			
Wednesday			
Thursday			
Friday			
Saturday			

Month 5 _____, Week 4

OBSERVATIONS

Wellness Calendar

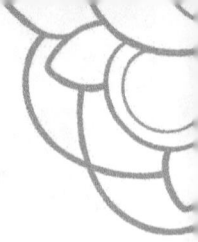

DAY	NIYAMA	ASANA	MEDITATION
Sunday			
Monday			
Tuesday			
Wednesday			
Thursday			
Friday			
Saturday			

Month 5 _____, Week 5

OBSERVATIONS

6
Classical Yoga

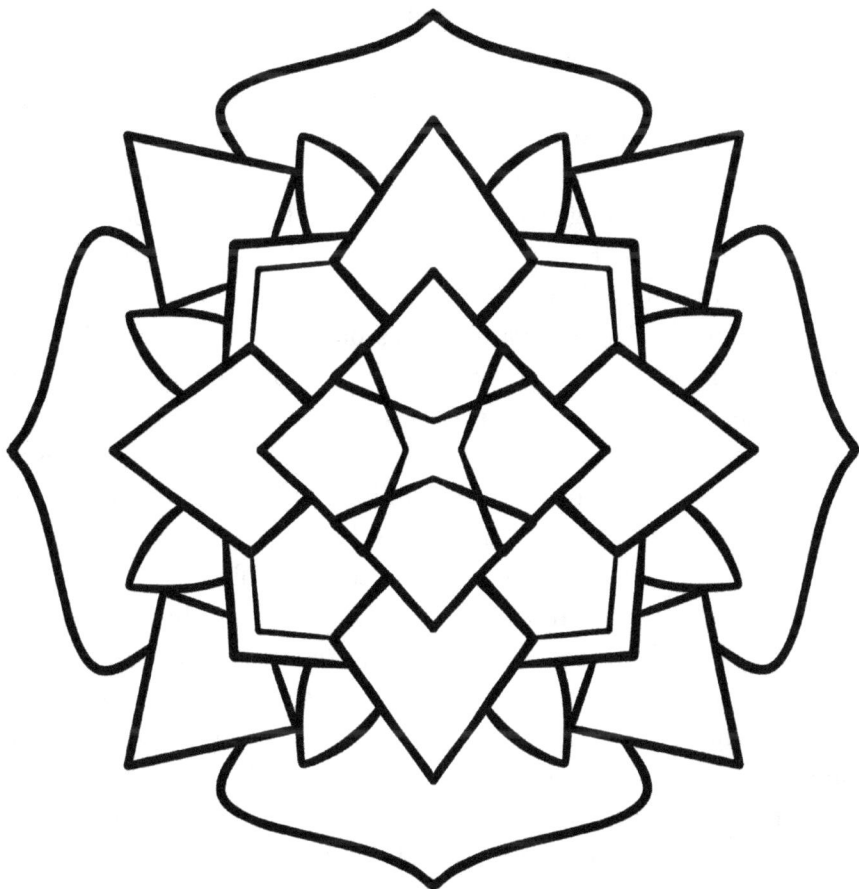

The Philosophy

"Being spiritual has nothing to do with what you believe
and everything to do with your state of consciousness."

— Eckhart Tolle

Classical yoga is a system of spiritual knowledge passed down from teachers with the most notable being Patanjali's Yoga Sutras. The sutras highlight the yoga philosophy with the *Eight Limbs of Yoga.*

Each of the limbs is sequenced to help the practitioner live a life of right and conscious action, and to help create an external and internal environment for spiritual growth and understanding. Right actions tend to have collective and individual benefits and help us stay connected both to self and to others. As humans, we are inter-related beings who rely and depend on each other for life. All great accomplishments of society have happened with shared humanity and shared purpose.

The eight limbs of yoga are steps designed in a particular order to prepare us for the next levels of a more conscious life and conscious living. Each step level is in preparation for the ultimate goal of Samadhi, mastery of the mind. The Eight Limb philosophy begins with accepting responsibility for our actions, continues with methods to help concentrate the fluctuating mind, and finally prepares us to live in a state of connection and bliss.

In this chapter, each aspect of the yoga philosophy is outlined. The first four limbs are followed by reflection questions that help personalize the yoga philosophy. My wish for you is to use each of the principles to create a prosperous life — one that supports you and the people around you.

Patanjali's *Eight Limbs of Yoga* are designed to guide us to a greater connection with ourselves at the deeper levels. For many of us, the connection to the innate self is made more challenging by the distractions and dramas of life. The guidelines highlight disciplined practices to help us connect to the deeper place within self: with Source, Love, the Universe and Consciousness. These are all words and concepts pointing us in the direction.

The following is an exercise to help outline the yoga philosophy along with guided reflections.

Self-Reflection Journaling 1

1. *Yama* is about our attitude towards our environment — being of service to others, treating all our surroundings with respect, love, and compassion.

Part 1: Take a moment to reflect on your attitude towards the environment. Reflect on your lifestyle and how you positively or (negatively) affect your environment, the air, soil, and levels of pollution. Write your reflections. What can you do to improve your effects on Mother Earth: the planet that supports us?

Part 2: Do you help the people around you whether they are family members, friends, or strangers? What can you do to help in any way? This can be as simple as smiling to strangers and connecting to them as if they are friends and loved ones.

2. *Niyama* is about our attitude toward ourselves. This includes treating ourselves with respect, love, and compassion, and taking care of our own physical, mental, and emotional well-being.

Take a moment to reflect on how you treat yourself and recognize "self-talk". Notice the commentary towards yourself in your mind. First, how often do you act on taking care of your physical body, your emotional and mental state? Taking care of the physical body may be through yoga and other forms of exercise. Taking care of your mental and emotional state may be with meditation and therapy or counseling.

Part 1: Wake up each morning and tell yourself *you love you.* If this is difficult, then begin with telling yourself that *you see you.* As you practice, make sure you are saying these words genuinely and with heart. It will get easier. Keep in mind that all our behaviors and actions begin on the inside. Learn to be kind to yourself. If you are kind to yourself, you may become more kind and loving to the people around you. If you are more compassionate with yourself, it's more likely you will be compassionate with the people around you. If you love yourself, you will be more loving with the people around you. Write down your experience noticing your self-talk, both positive and negative. Also, notice any discomfort around positive self-talk and self-nurturing.

Part 2: Use the *Niyama* column of your calendar and write down how you will take care of yourself each day. Begin the day with telling yourself *you love you* or *you see you.* Write down all the *activities* you plan on doing for yourself, including time for yourself to do yoga and meditation, therapy or counseling, get a massage or spend time in nature.

Make this part of the calendar and a part of your daily/weekly life. Investment in yourself for optimal health will result in a better investment in the world around you. How we treat ourselves will directly affect the way we treat the people and the world around us. Write down your reflections during weeks that you schedule time for activities you enjoy.

3. *Asana* is the physical practice of conditioning the body. It includes respecting the body by taking care of flexibility, strength, and overall health.

This limb is your *Asana,* or physical yoga practice. The practice of stretching and strengthening the body reinforces health and appreciation for the body. This is a reminder to nurture and respect the body for all that it does. Especially with injuries, illnesses, and the aging process, we continue to care for our body. The body is designed to heal, so we reinforce and promote the healing process.

Some of the tension in our body is blocked emotion, so don't be surprised when poses and/or stretches release this "built-up" energy.

Refer to the *Asana* column of the calendar:

Write down observations on each practice day including strength, flexibility, energy levels, improvements, changes, pains, and sensations.

You may also indicate the pose(s) where you felt more strength, flexibility, or balance?

Reflect on overall conditioning of the body. How does this reinforce self-care? How does this help set a path for self-observations? How does your physical practice help you connect deeper within?

_____

_____

_____

_____

_____

_____

_____

_____

_____

_____

_____

4. *Pranayama*, is restraint or expansion of the breath. It involves learning to observe, respect and understand the connection of the breath with the mind and the body.

Our life source is *Prana*, breath. Breath work on its own or as part of yoga and meditation practice is the most direct connection to the deeper self and to consciousness. Pranayama helps pause the perpetual thinking mind and brings us into the present moment. The practice takes focus and improves concentration.

A basic breathing technique is to count the breaths. Make the count a soft whisper in your head. Try each of these for 3–8 rounds.

    a. Inhale for 3 counts and exhale for 3 counts
    b. Inhale for 5 counts and exhale for 5 counts
    c. Inhale up to 8 counts and exhale for 8 counts

Reflect on the *experience* of the practice and the *results* of the practice on the mental and physical level. Write down where it may have felt easier and where it seemed more challenging.

Recognize the concentration and focus that is needed. Write down the effect on the thinking mind. Did it help you surrender to thinking to focus on your breathing? How?

Pranayama breathing techniques are attainable for all people, but they take focus, patience, and discipline. Breathing techniques help with levels of concentration, energize the body, calm the nervous system, and help detoxify the body.

5. *Pratyahara,* which translates to sense withdrawal. The withdrawal of the senses is the mental practice of not reacting to stimuli. This practice is in preparation for meditation and settling the mind.

This practice is challenging and is one that is further developed each time we meditate or practice. Whether we practice asana or meditation, we focus on a prolonged session and notice the distractions may be from the outside and/or from the inside. We notice that distractions come and go and so do thoughts. Sustained focus leads to improved concentration.

6. *Dharana* is concentration. Learning to concentrate has become more imperative in our distracting world.

This limb is closely connected to the prior. They are inter-related, as are all the *Eight Limbs.* Observation and concentration in our practice clears the way for a deeper connection, a spiritual practice.

7. *Dhyana,* which is meditation. The act of meditating brings the mental and physical benefits of calming the nervous system, lowering blood pressure, and working towards a clearer and stronger mind.

This limb helps us with resilience. Meditation is a practice of resilience. We learn to start over again and again. This takes practice, patience, and discipline. We condition the mind until we surrender to stillness and liberation from thought.

8. *Samadhi* is the complete integration of all limbs of yoga philosophy. Samadhi is the final step to becoming fully connected, self-realized, and self-aware. Samadhi is mastery of the mind.

As a witness to our own thinking minds, we soon recognize that our suffering is connected to our thoughts and beliefs. Mastery of the mind is the ability to let go of the thinking mind, the belief systems, and sometimes the lies that we cling to throughout our lives. These concepts cause much of our suffering, and the suffering continues with belief in false ideas.

Yoga philosophy is a way of life. It guides us in creating a nurturing environment with a more conscious, a more aware perspective. It leads us towards a life that supports others, our environment and ourselves. Following the path, we discover ourselves at the deepest level. When we function from this space, we can serve ourselves, each other, Planet Earth, and all living beings from a connected space. The connected space is consciousness itself.

Notes:

MONTH 6 WELLNESS CALENDAR

Schedule Hatha Yoga Practice 5 days per week
Schedule a 10-minute Meditation 5 days per week.

Wellness Calendar

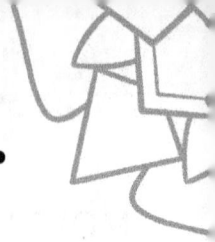

DAY	NIYAMA	ASANA	MEDITATI
Sunday			
Monday			
Tuesday			
Wednesday			
Thursday			
Friday			
Saturday			

Month 6 _____, Week 1

OBSERVATIONS

Wellness Calendar

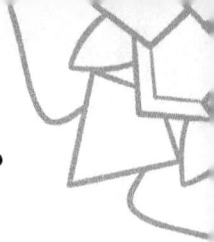

DAY	NIYAMA	ASANA	MEDITATION
Sunday			
Monday			
Tuesday			
Wednesday			
Thursday			
Friday			
Saturday			

Month 6 _____, Week 2

OBSERVATIONS

Wellness Calendar

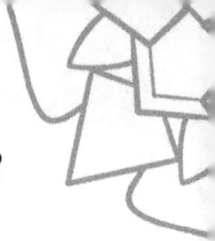

DAY	NIYAMA	ASANA	MEDITATION
Sunday			
Monday			
Tuesday			
Wednesday			
Thursday			
Friday			
Saturday			

Month 6 _____, Week 3

OBSERVATIONS

Wellness Calendar

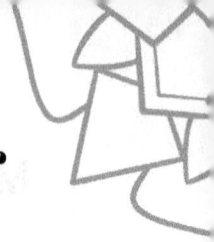

DAY	NIYAMA	ASANA	MEDITATI
Sunday			
Monday			
Tuesday			
Wednesday			
Thursday			
Friday			
Saturday			

Month 6 _____, Week 4

OBSERVATIONS

Wellness Calendar

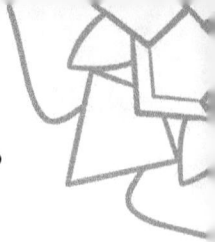

DAY	NIYAMA	ASANA	MEDITATION
Sunday			
Monday			
Tuesday			
Wednesday			
Thursday			
Friday			
Saturday			

Month 6 _____, Week 5

OBSERVATIONS

Sequence 3
40-Minute Vinyasa Flow

1. **Beginning Breathing:** Begin seated comfortably on the floor in easy pose.
   - Inhale and reach the arms out to the side and overhead. Exhale, turn the palms outward and float the arms down. Repeat 5 times.

2. **Seated Side Stretch:** Begin seated with the legs in easy pose.
   - Reach the right arm out to the side and place it on the floor and extend the left arm out and overhead and reach towards the right for a side body stretch. Repeat on the other side.

3. **Seated Easy Spine Twist Stretch:** Begin in Easy Pose.
   - Place right hand behind you and place the left hand outside the right knee.
   - Inhale and lengthen the spine, exhale and twist gently by bringing the shoulder back and looking back.
   - Hold for 3 breaths. Repeat on the left side.

4. **Cat/Cow:** Begin on hands and knees, or Tabletop position.
   - Place the hands directly below the shoulders and the knees directly below the hips.
   - Inhale and arch the spine looking up, exhale and round the spine looking towards the belly.
   - Repeat 3 times.

5. **Bird Dog:** Begin on hands and knees, or Tabletop position.
   - Engage the abdominal muscles.
   - Extend the right arm forward with right hand at the level of the right shoulder.
   - Extend the Left leg back with the foot flexed and in line with the left hip. Hold for 3 breaths. Repeat on the other side.

6. **Sun Salutation A (First Part Only – 2 rounds):** Begin from a standing position.
   - Inhale and reach the arms up overhead, pressing the palms together.
   - Exhale and bring the palms to heart center, round down and place hands on the floor.
   - Inhale and place the hands on the shins or knees and lift the torso halfway up.
   - Exhale and fold over the legs.
   - Inhale and come back up to standing position. Repeat salutation.

7. **Sun Salutation A (2 rounds):** Begin from a standing position.
   - Inhale and reach the arms up overhead, pressing the palms together.
   - Exhale and bring the palms to heart center, round down and place hands on the floor.
   - Inhale and place the hands on shins or knees and lift the torso halfway up.
   - Exhale and step back into a high plank and lower the body to the floor.
   - Inhale and lift the torso up into a low cobra pose.
   - Exhale and press the body up and back into Downward Facing Dog pose. Hold for 3 breaths. Repeat salutation.

8. Sun Salutation B: Begin from a standing position.
- Inhale. With the feet together, bend the knees and extend the arms up.
- Exhale and forward fold, placing hands on the floor and then lift the hips up.
- Inhale and gently place the hands on shins or knees and lift the torso halfway up.
- Exhale and step back into a high plank, then lower body down to the floor.
- Inhale and lift into a low cobra pose or Upward Facing Dog.
- Exhale and press back into Downward Facing Dog Pose.
- Inhale and lift the right leg up into Three-Legged Dog.

9. Warrior 1 Pose: Begin from the Downward Facing Dog position.
- Exhaling, step the right foot between the hands and bend the front knee. Keep the back heel on the floor with the back leg straight as you reach the arms up. Maintain proper hip alignment by gently pulling the right hip back and left hip forward. Hold for 3 Breaths.
- Inhale, and on the exhale, move into Warrior 2 Pose by bringing the right foot toward the center of the mat and adjust the left foot so that you see the front toe and heel of the right foot line up with the arch of the left foot. Bend the front knee so that the front leg creates a 90-degree angle. Keep the shoulders directly over the hips and gaze over the right hand. Hold for 3 Breaths.
- Inhale, and on the exhale, move into Extended Side Angle Pose by pivoting at the hip joint. Gently place the right elbow on the knee and reach the left arm up and over so that the left arm and the left leg create one straight line. Avoid leaning into the elbow. Hold for 3 Breaths.
- Inhale, and on the exhale, move into Reverse Warrior Pose by reaching the right arm straight up. Gaze up while gently placing the left hand on the left thigh or knee. Avoid placing weight in the left hand.

Keep the hips down with a deep bend in the front knee. Hold for 3 Breaths.

- From Downward Facing Dog repeat on the left side.

10. **Pigeon Pose:** Begin from Downward Facing Dog or on hands and knees.
    - Bend the right knee and place the right knee on the floor behind the right thumb. Position the right foot towards the middle line of the body and flex the right foot.
    - Extend the left leg back and slowly lower the hips down to the floor. Slowly bring your forearms and chest down to the floor and hold for 3 Breaths. Repeat with the Left Leg.

11. **Downward Boat:** Begin lying on the belly.
    - Separate the legs slightly and place the hands next to the hips on the floor.
    - Inhale and lift the upper body, arms and legs up while keeping the back of the neck long. Hold for 3 Breaths.

12. **Floor Bow:** Begin lying facedown.
    - Place the chin on the floor.
    - Bend both legs and grab the feet from the outside between the toes and heels.
    - Engage the gluteus muscles and actively kick the legs back and up while lifting the chest up. Hold for 3 Breaths.

13. **Child's Pose:** Sit with the hips on the heels.
    - Bring the big toes together and open the knees. Bend forward until your forehead touches the floor.
    - Press the hips back towards the heels and reach the arms forward. Hold for 3–5 Breaths.

14. **Camel Pose:** Kneel up on the knees and place the hands on the back of the hips (glutes).
    - Lift the chest and slowly move into a backbend.
    - Carefully work to grab the heels with the hands.
    - Maintain position of the hips directly over the knees.

15. **Bridge Pose:** Begin lying on your back.
    - Bend the knees placing the feet hip-width distance.
    - Slowly lift the hips up, then the middle back and chest while keeping the shoulders and the back of the head on the floor.
    - Press the feet downward, press the hips upward and engage the gluteus muscles.
    - Hold for 3 breaths.

16. **Reclined Twist:** Begin lying on your back.
    - Bend the right leg, gently place the right foot on the left knee.
    - Extend the right arm out to the side with the hand at the level of the shoulder.
    - Place the left hand on the outside of the right knee and gently bring the right knee towards the left. Hold the twist for 3 Breaths. Repeat on the other side.

17. **Stretching** — One legged forward fold to twist to side stretch: Begin in a seated position.
    - Extend the right leg straight forward and bend the left leg inward. Inhale arms up and exhale to fold over the right leg. Hold for 3 Breaths.

- Inhale to bring the torso up, place the left hand behind you and place the right hand outside the left knee and gently twist to the left from the lower back up and look back last. Hold for 3 Breaths.
- Untwist and place the right hand on the inside of the right knee and reach the left arm up and alongside the head for a side body stretch. Hold for 3 Breaths. Repeat on the other side.

18. **Alternate Nostril Breathing:** Sit comfortably with a straight spine.
    - With your right thumb cover the right nostril and with a slight turn of the wrist, cover the left nostril with the pinky and ring finger.
    - The index and middle finger can be folded inward or placed against the middle of the forehead between the eyebrows.
    - Rest the left hand gently on the left thigh.
    - To begin, cover your right nostril and inhale slowly through the left nostril for a count of 4.
    - Hold your breath and both nostrils briefly.
    - Release the right nostril only and exhale out for a count of 4.
    - Follow this immediately by inhaling through the right nostril; hold briefly and exhale out the left nostril for a count of 4.
    - This completes 1 Cycle. Continue for 3 more cycles with eyes closed.
    - Upon completion lower the right hand down to the right thigh and observe your breathing.
      * *This breathing lowers the blood pressure, balances the breath through the nostrils and calms the nervous system.*

7

Modern Yoga

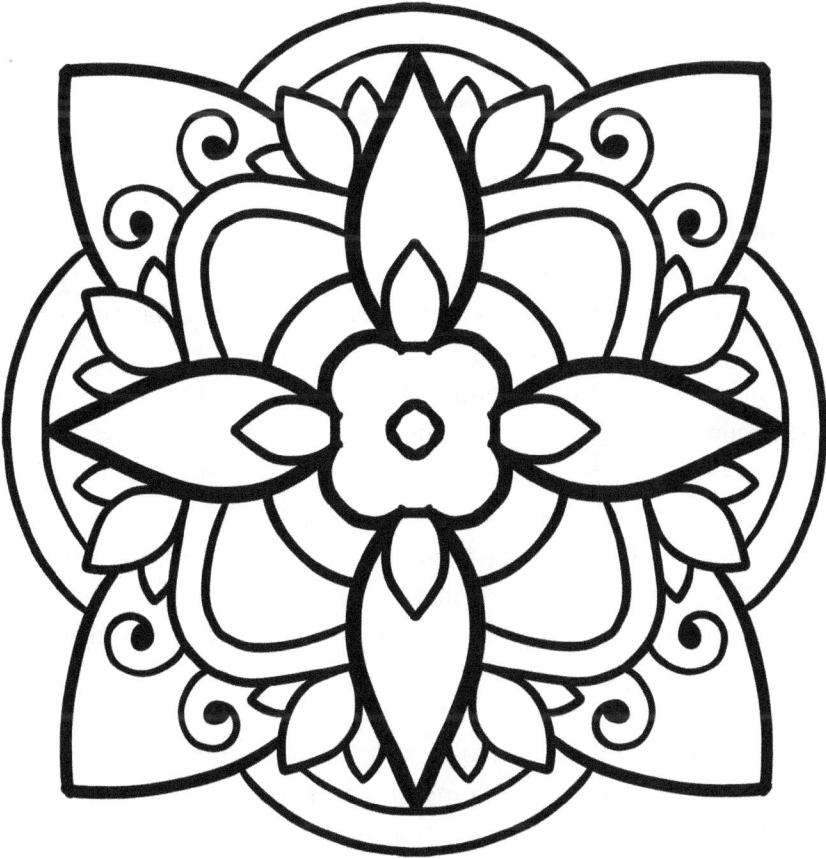

What is it and how was it influenced?

"Be aware of your breathing. Notice how this takes
attention away from your thinking and creates space."

— *Eckhart Tolle*

Modern yoga has sprung from a multitude of different backgrounds and styles and is generally considered the current day Vinyasa Yoga. Vinyasa is also known as *flow yoga,* which refers to the movement of the body with the breath. Vinyasa stems from the Krishnamacharya lineage. Krishnamacharya was a twentieth century Indian teacher who was referred to as "The Father of Modern Yoga." He was an influential yoga teacher who helped foster Pattabhi Jois and Ashtanga yoga, B.K.S. Iyengar, and Indra Devi. Modern yoga was also influenced by the Dutch and British colonization of India, which contributed to sequences that incorporate push-ups and planks called Sun Salutations.

Although most people in the West seek out yoga classes for strength or flexibility, the mental discipline of yoga is being neglected. Many of today's classes include music along with other additions that do not support the intended disciplinary practice. In this chapter, I would like you to experiment with a Vinyasa or any Hatha Yoga practice to recognize the focus and concentration needed. I encourage you to compare a practice using music and to notice the effect on your attention to breath and body sensations. The less external distractions we have in our practice, the more we tune into the messages in our body. Keep in mind that a Hatha, Vinyasa, or any Asana practice is intended to prepare you for more challenging practices of concentration, meditation, and insight.

As outlined in earlier chapters, Hatha Yoga and Asana practice require awareness just like a meditation practice. Since our brain's "attention" works like a flashlight, it is helpful to create an environment for focus and concentration. Our attention capability, just like a flashlight, is ineffective when scattered beyond a specific area.

Notice when your attention and presence practice becomes stronger, often you appreciate quieter environments. You may notice the fluctuations in your mind more clearly. You may also be more tuned into the breath, thought patterns and surroundings.

Although I recommend avoiding music with most of your practice, I invite you to experience the effects of music on your own. Below, I have outlined a few key points to pay attention to so you may observe and compare the difference in a practice with and without music.

Vinyasa Practice *without* Music

- Stay with the breath.

- Listen to the body.

- Stay focused and present.

- Make note of focus, connection, and concentration levels in your practice.

Vinyasa Practice *with* Music

- Stay with the breath: Was the breath secondary to the music?

- Listen to the body: Was it more or less challenging to pay full attention to the sensations of the body?

- Stay focused and present: Did the music take you to a different moment in time or event? Was the mind fluctuating more or less? Make note of focus and concentration levels of your practice.

MONTH 7 CALENDAR

Schedule Vinyasa Yoga Practice 5 days per week.

Schedule a 5-minute Meditation 5–7 times per week.

Wellness Calendar

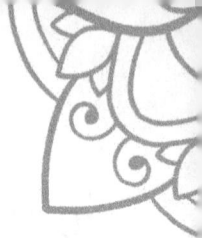

DAY	NIYAMA	ASANA	MEDITATIO
Sunday			
Monday			
Tuesday			
Wednesday			
Thursday			
Friday			
Saturday			

Month 7 _____, Week 1

OBSERVATIONS

Wellness Calendar

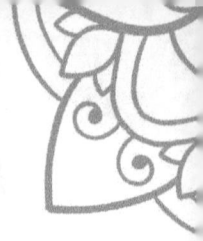

DAY	NIYAMA	ASANA	MEDITATI
Sunday			
Monday			
Tuesday			
Wednesday			
Thursday			
Friday			
Saturday			

Month 7 _____, Week 2

OBSERVATIONS

Wellness Calendar

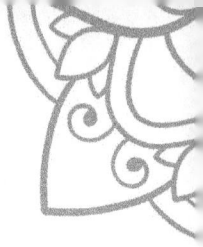

DAY	NIYAMA	ASANA	MEDITATION
Sunday			
Monday			
Tuesday			
Wednesday			
Thursday			
Friday			
Saturday			

Month 7 _____, Week 3

OBSERVATIONS

Wellness Calendar

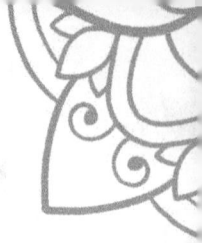

DAY	NIYAMA	ASANA	MEDITATIO
Sunday			
Monday			
Tuesday			
Wednesday			
Thursday			
Friday			
Saturday			

Month 7 _____, Week 4

OBSERVATIONS

Wellness Calendar

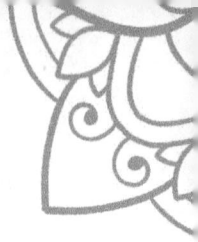

DAY	NIYAMA	ASANA	MEDITATI
Sunday			
Monday			
Tuesday			
Wednesday			
Thursday			
Friday			
Saturday			

Month 7 _____, Week 5

OBSERVATIONS

8
Yoga Today

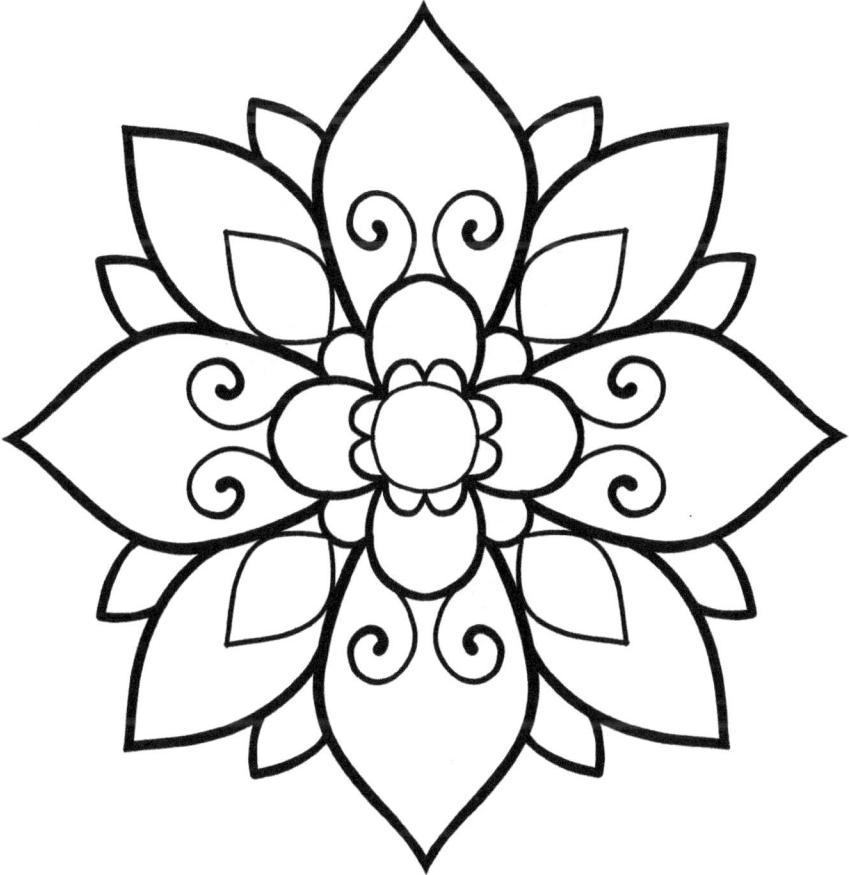

The Direction of Yoga and Meditation

"Most of us are accustomed to looking outside of ourselves for fulfillment. We are living in a world that conditions us to believe that outer attainments can give us what we want. Yet again and again our experiences show us that nothing external can completely fulfill the deep longing within for something more."

— *Paramahansa Yogananda*

Many of today's yoga classes have no resemblance to yoga except for the poses. The essential component of yoga as meditation and connection is watered-down or lost. As mentioned earlier, people seek out yoga for different reasons that usually have to do with better overall health. As our society is learning quickly, better health is not just physical but most of it is mental and emotional.

In the last couple of years dealing with the Global Pandemic, many people turned to meditation and yoga for the mental and emotional benefits and are now beginning to understand the deeper levels of the practice. The challenges we encountered recently led us to plunge deeper, to connect to ourselves, and to seek comfort and safety within our own mind and body rather than the outside world. In this chapter, I would like you to take notice of various external distractions that remove you from a peaceful and calm state. Notice how outside influences remove you from a deeper connection to self. Our yoga and meditation practice can be considered our sanctuary for healing, where we eliminate distractions to settle into serenity, create space and invite calm into our lives. This is necessary for our health, our nervous system, and overall well-being.

Many anxiety and depressive disorders come from too much focus on the outside world, where meditation and yoga help us to tune into our inner world. This inner world is where we connect to the deeper self. The deeper self is unchanging. The deeper self does not "need" anything from the outside world to be whole.

It's important to create a space for ourselves to eliminate all distractions. Creating space for ourselves may include practicing yoga, meditation, or simply sitting still and observing nature. When we eliminate distractions and noise, there are less fluctuations in the mind. When the mind is not distracted with stories that are ultimately irrelevant to us, we tend to be more grounded in reality.

The reality that helps ground us is not the reality of our thoughts. The thoughts are what bring us suffering. The reality that grounds us is what is happening right now, in this space, with the breath, and in the present moment. When dealing with life's challenges, the mind is overactive, fluctuating, worrying, doubting, and the emotions get dragged through some dark places. When we are dealing with a major life challenge such as illness, loss, or conflict, we are best served by bringing our thoughts back to the present moment. It is a simple yet challenging practice.

For example, right now, my problems only exist in my mind and are based on past or future events. Neither the past nor the future exists *right now*. They are both only thoughts and stories in my head. Right now, I am sitting at my desk in a warm home with my feet on the ground, my lungs taking the breath in and my attention on writing this sentence. This is the present moment. I am consciously working and staying with each moment as it unfolds. In my mind, I'm not partially in the past or partially in the future. Neither exists anywhere but in the mind.

Presence practice, awareness practice, yoga and meditation can all be done in the comfort of your own home daily. With self-observation you are continually directed back to your deeper self. You are empowering yourself with practices that reinforce the deeper unchanging self. Yoga and meditation practices guide you back to yourself and your Home within.

Self-reflection Journaling 1

What adjustments can you make or have you made to create a happier life — physically, mentally, and emotionally?

Can you reduce the distractions in your daily life by reducing social media? Do you recognize that advertising and media serve as more noise? Do you sometimes seek distractions? If so, why?

_____

_____

_____

_____

_____

_____

_____

_____

_____

Self-reflection Journaling 2

Upon incorporating healthy habits, yoga, and meditation, do you feel stronger physically? Clearer mentally? More stable emotionally? If not, what can you do to reinforce these key elements of your well-being?

_____

_____

_____

_____

_____

_____

_____

_____

_____

_____

_____

_____

Self-reflection Journaling 3

What does connecting to the Self mean for you? Do you feel a strong connection to the deeper self? Do you feel a disconnect from your deeper self, if so, why? How can you change this or incorporate practices such as stillness, yoga, meditation, or prayer to connect deeper? Has your connection to the deeper self-improved with regular yoga and meditation practices?

_____

_____

_____

_____

_____

_____

_____

_____

_____

_____

_____

Self-reflection Journaling 4

What does *peace* feel like to you and what needs to happen for you to feel it? Do you have any control of external events that bring you peace? If so, how?

Do you have control over your peace from within? How do the effects of yoga and meditation practice help this process? How do your practices bring you closer to this feeling of peace?

MONTH 8 CALENDAR

Schedule Vinyasa or Hatha Yoga Practice 5 days per week

Schedule a 10-Minute Meditation 5 days per week

Wellness Calendar

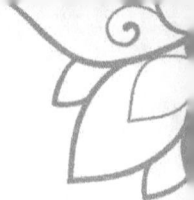

DAY	NIYAMA	ASANA	MEDITATION
Sunday			
Monday			
Tuesday			
Wednesday			
Thursday			
Friday			
Saturday			

Month 8 _____, Week 1

OBSERVATIONS

Wellness Calendar

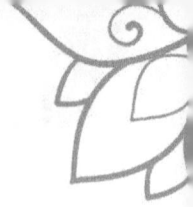

DAY	NIYAMA	ASANA	MEDITATI
Sunday			
Monday			
Tuesday			
Wednesday			
Thursday			
Friday			
Saturday			

Month 8 _____, Week 2

OBSERVATIONS

Wellness Calendar

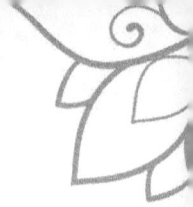

DAY	NIYAMA	ASANA	MEDITATION
Sunday			
Monday			
Tuesday			
Wednesday			
Thursday			
Friday			
Saturday			

Month 8 _____, Week 3

OBSERVATIONS

Wellness Calendar

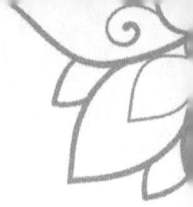

DAY	NIYAMA	ASANA	MEDITATI
Sunday			
Monday			
Tuesday			
Wednesday			
Thursday			
Friday			
Saturday			

Month 8 _____, Week 4

OBSERVATIONS

Wellness Calendar

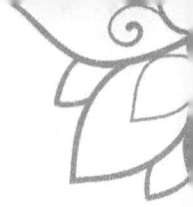

DAY	NIYAMA	ASANA	MEDITATIO
Sunday			
Monday			
Tuesday			
Wednesday			
Thursday			
Friday			
Saturday			

Month 8 _____, Week 5

OBSERVATIONS

9
Our Compass

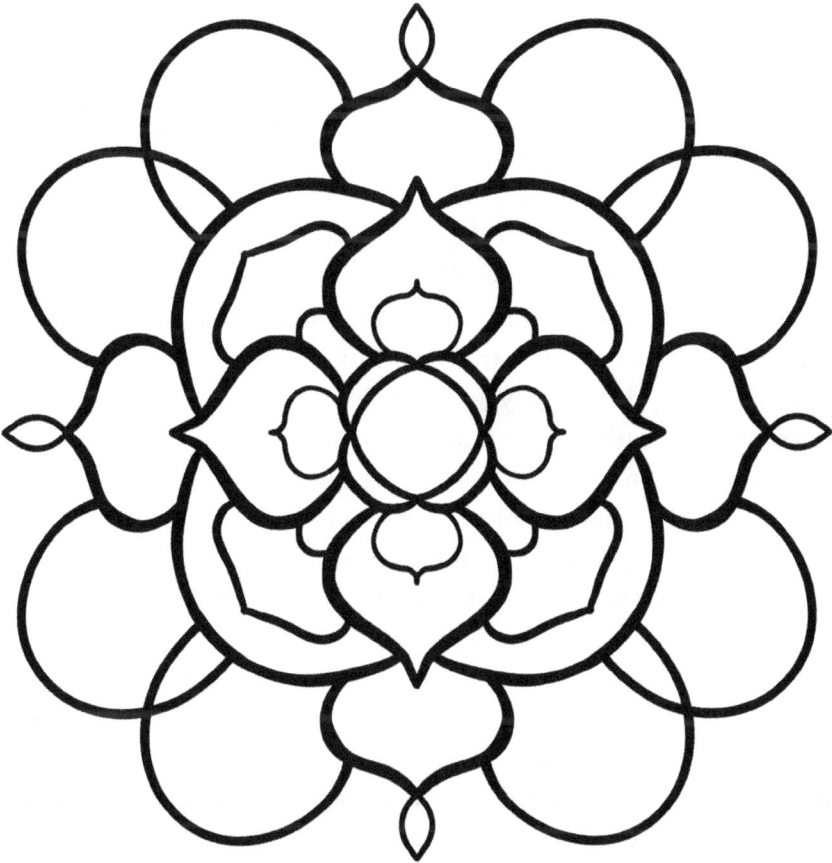

How to Get Back on the Path

"Yesterday I was clever, so I wanted to change the World.
Today I am wise, so I am changing myself."

— *Rumi*

For some people, the physical benefits of yoga may be enough. Yet for many of us who seek a life of self-reflection, self-healing, and deeper connection...we want more, and there is more. The initial steps of yoga set us on the path. What is the path? The path is following practices to help recognize there is more to us than the physical body. There is the deeper self, the conscious self that is part of the Universe, part of Source, part of Divinity or God. It does not matter what the word or concept is. What matters is to feel it and be tuned into it, to know that we are whole at our core and to learn to trust our internal guide. Yet, to "hear" the internal guide, we must quiet the external and internal noise.

It takes dedication to oneself to practice the discipline of self-observation and self-reflection. Yoga philosophy supports this by highlighting principles that help us and the people around us. In this chapter, I would like for you to recognize that the work we do on ourselves and within is the catalyst for true change.

Self-reflection and self-observation are key to understanding our mental and emotional health. Through honest observations of self, we recognize triggers that magnify our suffering and unhappiness. Instead of *being* our thoughts and actions, we learn to *observe* our thoughts and actions. This shift in perspective helps create space from habits and traumas that may bring us recurring misery and pain.

To connect to the deeper self, we need to remove the mental noise, belief systems and habits that keep us from recognizing the deep presence within. We are constantly stimulated, triggered, and often pommeled by outside noise and influence. First, we need to learn skills to ground ourselves, such as practices like yoga and meditation. Next, we become aware of our thoughts, actions, and behaviors. With the right action, we learn to take responsibility for ourselves, eliminating victim identity and blame. With responsibility for ourselves, actions, and thoughts, we begin self-reflection. We first observe, and then reflect, and start our process to seek deeper levels. Once you "know" yourself, learn to be kind and compassion-ate towards yourself. In the process, learn to love yourself and you will find a greater sense of peace.

Karma is a reality of life. ALL our actions have consequences. With meditation and yoga, we practice silence. We learn to slow down and approach life in new or improved ways. We listen deeper within. This can rarely be experienced with just one yoga or med-itation practice. The long-term results are in the repetition. We re-inforce our mental, emotional, and physical health to help us move through the challenges that come our way.

Mental and emotional health is key in leading a peaceful and happy life. Regular reinforcement of mental and emotional health practices allow us to recover more quickly after stressful events and challenges. We improve our resilience and strength not just physi-cally, but mentally, emotionally, and spiritually as well.

Self-reflection Journaling 1

What do you seek in daily practice of yoga and meditation?

Upon completion of a yoga or meditation practice, what is true for you? What is your wish, your prayer or deepest desire?

Can you witness the inner stillness, the witnessing presence, the deeper self? How important is it for you to tap into this?

_____

_____

_____

_____

_____

_____

_____

_____

_____

_____

_____

_____

_____

_____

_____

_____

_____

_____

Self-reflection Journaling 2

Imagine your wish or deepest desire is fulfilled, will this change you as a person within yourself and to the outside world? If so, how?

_____

_____

_____

_____

_____

_____

_____

_____

_____

Self-reflection Journaling 3

Keep Karma in mind; everything we do has consequence. We are inter-related beings.

How do you want to be remembered as a person? With your actions?

How do you feel this wish or desire will benefit the people around you?

_____

_____

_____

_____

_____

_____

_____

_____

_____

_____

_____

_____

_____

_____

MONTH 9 CALENDAR

Schedule Yoga Practice 5 days per week.
Schedule a 5-minute Meditation 5 days per week.

Wellness Calendar

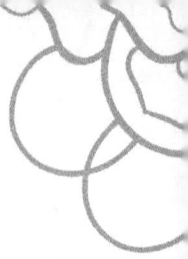

DAY	NIYAMA	ASANA	MEDITATI
Sunday			
Monday			
Tuesday			
Wednesday			
Thursday			
Friday			
Saturday			

Month 9 _____, Week 1

OBSERVATIONS

Wellness Calendar

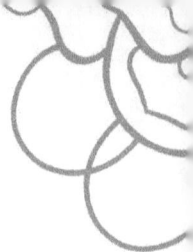

DAY	NIYAMA	ASANA	MEDITATIO
Sunday			
Monday			
Tuesday			
Wednesday			
Thursday			
Friday			
Saturday			

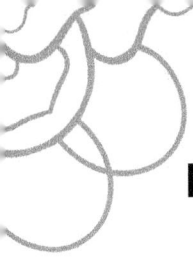

Month 9 _____, Week 2

OBSERVATIONS

Wellness Calendar

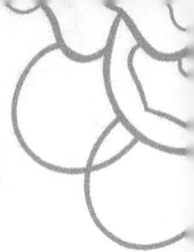

DAY	NIYAMA	ASANA	MEDITATIO
Sunday			
Monday			
Tuesday			
Wednesday			
Thursday			
Friday			
Saturday			

Month 9 _____, Week 3

OBSERVATIONS

Wellness Calendar

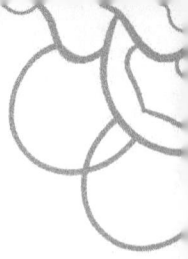

DAY	NIYAMA	ASANA	MEDITATION
Sunday			
Monday			
Tuesday			
Wednesday			
Thursday			
Friday			
Saturday			

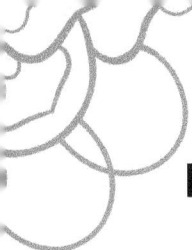

Month 9 _____, Week 4

OBSERVATIONS

Wellness Calendar

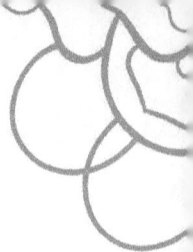

DAY	NIYAMA	ASANA	MEDITATIO
Sunday			
Monday			
Tuesday			
Wednesday			
Thursday			
Friday			
Saturday			

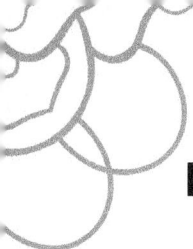

Month 9 _____, Week 5

OBSERVATIONS

Sequence 4
40-Minute Intermediate Practice

STANDING POSES

1. **Standing Deep Breathing:** Begin with feet together or slightly apart.
   - Interlace the fingers with palms together and place hands under the chin.
   - Simultaneously inhale by the nose through 6 counts, while lifting the elbows as high as possible.
   - Hold for 1 count.
   - Exhale by the mouth for 6 counts, gently tilting the head back while bringing elbows forward and together.
   - Repeat for a total of 8 Breaths.

2. **Lunge:** Begin standing with feet together, place hands on hips.
   - Take a big step forward on the right foot and slowly bend the right knee.
   - Keep the back leg straight and lift the back heel until the heel is directly over the toes.
   - Be sure the right foot is directly ahead of the right hip.
   - Inhale arms up overhead and bring palms together.
   - Exhale and slowly move into a backbend by lifting the chest and bringing the arms back.
   - Hold for 3 Breaths. Repeat on the left side.

3. **Sun Salutation:** Begin in standing position.
   - Place the palms together at heart center.
   - Inhale, lift the arms up, and move into a standing backbend.
   - Exhale slowly, move into a forward bend, and place hands on the floor with the fingertips in line with the toes. Bring the forehead towards the knees.

- Bend the knees, and balance in a squat position with the knees together and the forehead touching the knees.
- Step the right leg back and then the left leg and hold in Plank Position.
- Lower the body down to the floor and lift the chest into a low Cobra Pose.
- Press back into Downward Facing Dog and hold for 3 Breaths.
- Step the right foot forward and then the left and move back into a squat with the forehead to the knees.
- Lift the hips up and keep the forehead touching the knees.
- Round up with palms in prayer and reach the arms up at the top and move into a standing backbend.
- End with palms in prayer position.

STANDING HALF MOON POSE WITH BACKBEND AND HANDS TO FEET POSE

1. **Half Moon:** Begin standing with feet together or slightly apart.
   - Inhale and reach the arms up overhead.
   - Bring the palms together and cross the thumbs.
   - Inhale and extend the upper body to the right.
   - Maintain equal weight in the feet and keep the legs and arms in straight positions.
   - Keep the chest open.
   - Hold for 3 breaths. Repeat on the other side.

Backbend
- Keep arms extended straight up and engage the gluteus muscles.
- Lift the chest and slowly move into a backbend. Find the depth where you can maintain the position and hold for 3 breaths.

Forward Bend to Hands-to-feet Pose
- Slowly move into a forward fold and grab the heels (or ankles).
- Connect the legs to the upper body and slowly straighten the legs and stretch the spine downward.
- Maintain upper and lower body connection and hold for 3 breaths.

2. **Triangle Pose:** Begin with the feet together.
   - Take a 5-foot step to the right, and stretch the arms to the sides so they are parallel to the floor.
   - Turn the right foot until it's parallel to the edge of the mat. Turn the left foot inward slightly.
   - Bend the right knee until the hip is at the level of the knee and the knee is directly over the right ankle. Maintain a straight left leg.
   - Move arms together and place the right elbow in front of the right knee while reaching the right arm downward. At the same time reach the left arm straight upward so that the arms together form one straight line.
   - Keep the lift hip forward slightly, bring the left shoulder back, and look up towards the palm of the left hand.
   - Hold for 3 breaths. Repeat on the left side.

3. **Separate Leg Forehead-to-knee Pose:** Begin standing with the feet together and the arms extended straight up with the palms together.
   - Take a 3-foot step to the right, and lift the toes and rotate on the heels so that the right foot is forward and the back foot is turned

at an angle. Keep the arms extended straight upward and palms together.

- Bring the chin down and slowly articulate the spine while rounding forward until the right knee touches the forehead while bending the knee towards the forehead to connect.
- Keep arms extended forward ahead of the right foot.
- Hold for 3 breaths. Repeat on the left side.

4. Chair Pose (3 parts):

Part I: Begin standing with feet hip-width distance.
- Inhale and reach the arms forward with palms facing down and arms straight.
- Exhale and bring the hips down until the hips are slightly above the knees.
- Hold for 3 Breaths.

Part II: Keep the feet hip-width distance and arms parallel to the floor.
- Lift the heels until the heels are over the toes.
- Contract the leg, glute and abdominal muscles and slowly bend the knees until the hips are slightly above the knees, maintaining the position of the heels directly over the toes.
- Hold for 3 breaths.

Part III, Classic Chair:
- Bring the feet and knees together.
- Lift the arms upward at an angle and sit the hips down. Keep the feet and knees together and hold for 3 breaths.

5. **Eagle Pose:** Begin with feet together and arms by the sides.
   - Inhale and reach the arms up overhead.
   - Exhale and bring the right arm under the left arm and wrap them around each other 1–2 times. Ideally, bring the palms together.
   - Bend the knees and bring the hips down and lift the right leg over the left leg and wrap the legs around 1–2 times. If possible, wrap the toes around the back of the ankle.
   - Hold the compression for 3 breaths and repeat on the left side.

6. **Standing Head-to-knee, Parts I, II, and III:** Begin standing with feet together.

   ### Part I
   - Interlace the fingers. Lift the right knee up in front and round the spine to hold the right foot in the hands. Hold the foot slightly ahead of the arch.
   - Keep the standing leg straight with the left thigh muscle contracted so that the left knee is fully extended.

   ### Part II
   - Slowly extend the right leg forward and maintain heel at the same level as the right hip. Keep the abdominal muscles contracted and the spine rounded. Extend the right leg until the knee is fully extended and the thigh contracted.
   - Keep both knees extended and both thighs contracted and the spine rounded.

   ### Part III
   - Keep both legs straight, with knees extended and thighs contracted. Bend the elbows down next to the calves, rounding the spine and hold for 3 Breaths. Repeat on the left side.

7. **Standing Bow:** Begin standing with feet together.
   - Bend the right knee back, lifting the foot up behind the body.
   - Hold the right foot from behind. Ideally, the palm is facing outward (avoid twisting the wrist).
   - Extend the left arm straight up towards the ceiling.
   - Begin pressing the right foot back into the hand to create a backbend.
   - Slowly bring the torso and upper body downward toward the floor. Hold for 3 Breaths. Repeat on the left side.

8. **Balancing Stick:** Begin standing with the feet together.
   - Inhale the arms straight up overhead and bring the palms together and cross the thumbs.
   - Step forward on the right foot and bring the upper body down and the left leg straight up behind you.
   - Maintain a straight line from the fingertips to the left toes. Work towards bringing the upper body and left leg parallel to the floor.
   - Hold for 3 Breaths and repeat on the left side.

9. **Separate Leg Stretching:** Begin standing with the feet together.
   - Take a wide 4–5 foot step to the side and position the feet so they are parallel to each other.
   - With arms extended out to the sides, bend forward at the hips and grab the heels. Straighten both legs so the knees are fully extended and the thighs are contracted.
   - Hold the feet at the heels and bend the elbows back towards the shins.
   - Touch the forehead to the floor and hold for 3 breaths.

10. **Tree Pose:** Begin standing with the feet together.
    - Lift the right knee in front of the body as high as possible and gently bring the right foot to the top of the left thigh.
    - Keep the standing leg straight. Contract the abdominal and gluteus muscles and stand tall. Hold for 3 breaths.

Sequence 4 *continued*

FLOOR

1. **Wind Removing Pose:** Begin in a reclined position.
    - Bend the right knee and hold below the knee with fingers interlaced.
    - Pull the knee towards the shoulder, thigh alongside the ribcage and hold for 3 Breaths. Repeat on the Left side.
    - Bend both knees up and keep the knees together.
    - Reach for the opposite elbows and pull both knees in while pressing the hips down towards the floor. Try to create an extended spine against the floor. Hold for 3 breaths.

2. **Cobra:** Begin lying on the stomach.
    - Place the palms underneath the chest with the fingertips in line with the top of the shoulders and the outer edge of the hands in line with the outer edges of the shoulders. Keep the legs straight and together with the tops of the feet against the floor.
    - Inhale and lift the upper body until the elbows create a 90-degree angle.
    - Hold for 3 breaths.

3. **Locust:** Begin lying on the stomach.
    - Place the chin on the floor and bring the arms into a straight position underneath the body, pointing towards the feet. The palms should be flat on the floor and the fingers spread out.
    - Inhale and lift the right leg up to 45-degrees. Keep the right hip against the right forearm. Continuously press both hands and shoulders against the floor. Hold for 3 breaths and repeat with the left leg.
    - Place the mouth on the floor. Inhale, engage the gluteus and leg muscles and lift both legs together. Keep the legs together, thighs contracted and feet touching. Hold for 3 breaths.

4. Full Locust: Lying on the stomach.
- Keep the legs together and active and reach the arms straight out to the sides with the palms downward.
- Contract all the muscles, including the gluteus, legs, and arms. At the same time, lift the upper body, arms, and legs off the floor.
- Hold for 3 breaths.

5. Bow Pose: Begin facedown with the chin on the floor.
- Bend both legs at the knees and grab the feet from the outside, halfway between the toes and heels.
- Engage the gluteus muscles, inhale, and actively kick the legs back and up. Hold for 3 breaths.

6. Child's Pose: Sit with the hips on the heels.
- Bring the big toes together and open the knees. Bend forward until your forehead touches the floor.
- Press the hips back towards the heels and reach the arms forward. Hold for 3–5 Breaths.

7. Half Tortoise: Sit with the hips on the heels.
- Inhale and extend the arms overhead with the palms together.
- Keep the arms and spine straight, and slowly hinge forward at the hips.
- Gently place the forehead on the floor and actively reach the arms forward.
- Keep the palms flat and pressing together, elbows extended, and simultaneously press the hips back towards the heels.
- Hold for 3–5 Breaths

8. **Camel Pose:** Kneel up on the knees and place the hands on the back of the hips (glutes).
   - Lift the chest and slowly move into a backbend.
   - Carefully work to grab the heels with the hands.
   - Maintain position of the hips directly over the knees.
   - This being the deepest backbend. Take a rest at this point by lying on your back in Savasana or sit with hips on heels and press palms together. Take 3–5 Breaths.

9. **Rabbit Pose:** Begin sitting on your heels with the feet together.
   - Grab the heels with the thumbs on the outside and the fingertips on the inside of the heels. Make sure you have a tight grip.
   - Contract the abdominal muscles, bring the chin down and slowly round your spine forward to bring the forehead to the knees.
   - Slowly lift the hips while simultaneously pulling on the heels. Avoid placing weight in the top of the head. Only a slight amount is safe. Keep the feet touching each other and against the floor and hold for 3 Breaths.

10. **Stretching Pose:** Begin in a seated position.
    - Extend the right leg out at an angle and bend the left leg.
    - Grab the right foot with both hands and connect the forehead to the knee.
    - Slowly straighten the right leg while maintaining forehead-to-knee connection.
    - With a rounded spine, begin bending the elbows down to touch the floor on either side of the calf. Hold for 3 breaths and repeat with the left leg.

    Straddle: Extend both legs out at an angle and keep the heels in the same line. Walk the hands forward while keeping the legs straight. Work towards maintaining a straight spine.

Hands to Feet: Bring the legs and feet together. Hook the big toes with the index and middle fingers. Work on straightening the legs and the spine. You may have to work on one at a time. Hold for 3 to 5 breaths.

11. **Spine Twist with Bent Legs:** Begin with both legs out in front.
    - Bend the right knee and place the right foot outside the left knee.
    - Bend the left knee and place the left foot outside the right hip. Make sure both sides of the hips are evenly on the floor.
    - Place the right hand behind you at the base of the spine.
    - Reach the left arm up and place the left elbow outside the right knee.
    - Inhale and lengthen the spine and exhale, twisting the spine from the lower back upward so that the head and neck turns last.
    - Hold for 3 breaths. Repeat on the left side.

12. **Kapalabhati Breathing (faster rhythm):** Sit comfortably with a straight spine.
    - Completely relax the abdominal muscles.
    - Visualize blowing out candles through pursed lips. Exhale and blow the imaginary candles out repeatedly for 50 counts at a steady pace. Contract the belly quickly on the exhale. If you are doing this correctly, the belly contracts back in order to force the breath out. Avoid focusing on the inhale. Exhale 50 times at a steady rhythm.

13. **Closing Meditation:** Stay seated upright or lie comfortable on your back with your eyes closed.
    - Focus on the flow of the breath.
    - Slowly scan your body from the head down to the feet and relax any remaining tension in the body.
    - Stay resting and observing the breath for as long as needed.

10
Self-Compassion

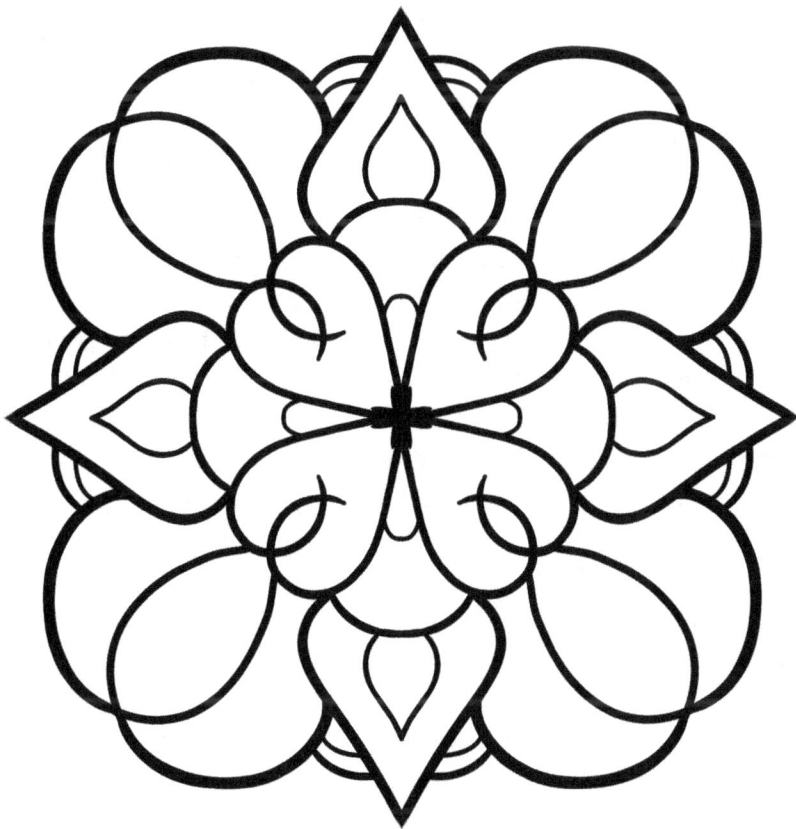

A True Art in Self-Care

"We speak about losing our minds as if it is a bad thing.
I say, lose your mind. Do it purposefully. Find out who you
really are beyond your thoughts and beliefs."

— *Vironika Tugaleva*

The meaning of compassion is *to suffer together*. Among emotion researchers, it is defined as the feeling that arises when you are confronted with another's suffering and feel motivated to relieve that pain. Although compassion is not the same as empathy, the two concepts are related. Empathy is the ability to understand and share the feelings of another and take their perspective. Yet, to have compassion, first you must notice that a person is hurting, then you feel moved by their anguish and finally, the heart responds to their pain. You feel warmth and caring and the desire to help end the suffering for that person in some way. It also means you offer understanding and kindness when the person makes a mistake rather than judging them harshly. Another important understanding of compassion is that it is not pity you feel for the other. You realize that suffering, failure, and imperfection are part of the **shared human experience**.

Self-compassion involves compassion towards yourself when you have a difficult time, fail, or notice something you don't like about yourself. Instead of just ignoring the pain with a stiff-upper-lip mentality, stop to ask yourself, "This is really difficult right now, how can I comfort and care for myself in this moment?"

In this chapter, I would like you to notice your behavior towards yourself in times you feel you made a mistake or failed somehow. Recognize your self-talk and actions that may be disconnected or abusive. Try to incorporate some more self-compassion and notice how this little pause and self-nurturing allows you to move past your challenge with more awareness.

This simple practice of taking a pause, acknowledging our pain, and giving ourselves comfort is a big step towards personal growth and self-healing. To take a moment to acknowledge our pain and nurture ourselves takes care of our inner world. When we push down or deny our hurt or our mistakes, it does not go away. A moment of acknowledgement allows for more self-love, which transfers to the World and people around us. Ultimately, our true home is created in our inner world, the home where we feel safe, nurtured, and comforted.

Below is a summary of the **RAIN** method introduced to me by Tara Brach. It was originally presented 20 years ago by Michele McDonald for mindfulness practice.

RAIN is an easy acronym for the following:

Recognize the situation. Ask yourself: "What is happening inside? What are the sensations/emotions?"

Allow life to be as it is. Allow for the discomfort to be there. Notice what is true in the moment and try not to push it away.

Investigate what the discomfort feels like. Do you feel tightness in the throat or chest or gut area?

Nurture yourself with loving presence and words such as "I know you're hurting."

Self-reflection Journaling 1

In what area of your life do you feel stuck? Do your actions continue to manifest the same results? Notice what your thoughts and belief systems may be. This is an area you may be able to *Awaken.* Become aware of your thoughts and actions. Become aware of your triggers. The areas of our lives that tend to trigger us emotionally are usually the areas we may want to invite more awareness.

Part 1: Write down the challenge (current or past).

Part 2: Answer this question: "Is this a recurring challenge in my life?"

Part 3: Investigate a little deeper. What is the root of this challenge? What is my belief about myself in this situation? Does it have to do with self-worth and how?

Part 4: Write down how you can take care of yourself with reminders of kindness and compassion.

Try to be impeccable in your words with the people around you and especially with yourself.

Self-reflection Journaling 2

Self-compassion includes being warm and understanding toward ourselves. As humans, we cannot always be or get exactly what we want. When this reality is denied or fought against, suffering increases in the form of stress, frustration, and self-criticism. When this reality is accepted with sympathy and kindness, greater emotional balance is experienced.

Part 1: With the clarification of self-compassion, think of a person you care deeply about. Write down a situation that caused this person suffering. What feelings and motivation prompted you to help this loved one?

What actions (if any) did you want to take to help?

Part 2: Imagine a moment when you are suffering or a time when you feel you have failed or felt inadequate. What do you do in this moment?

Do you shut down emotionally, feel embarrassment, shame or anger? Do you tend to reach for food, alcohol or shopping to comfort you?

How can you match your actions towards yourself to that of how you comforted your loved one? What actions (if any) would you take? What words would you say? Keep in mind, if this is still challenging for you, you may want to imagine your "future wise self" speaking to you, or someone who loves you and cares for you such as a parent, a grandparent, a mentor. You may even imagine someone who is no longer living that you love and admire.

_____

_____

_____

_____

_____

_____

_____

_____

_____

_____

Self-reflection Journaling 3

Suffering and personal inadequacy are part of the *shared human experience.* We all go through similar challenges in our lives, and it is important *not* to identify too closely with our specific difficulties. When this perspective is incorporated, the challenge is simply that — a challenge — not something that defines us. You become aware of it instead of being overtaken by it. Our challenges are here to wake us up. To help us understand that life will continue to test us, so we must learn to move through difficult times with more aware-ness, wisdom, and acknowledge a deeper connection to ourselves. Knowing, and more importantly, feeling, that we belong to some-thing larger than ourselves is the path towards home.

Part 1: Write down an event in your life that caused a lot of suffering.

Part 2: Now take a moment to reflect on others you may know who have gone through a similar challenge. If you do not personally know them, you may know *of* them. Write down their name and the challenge that you can relate to. It may be someone who experienced some kind of loss such as a relationship, a loved-one, a home, or a business. Conclude with the similarities between the challenge you personally had and this person's challenges. Sit with the fact that most people in this world have similar challenges and with the shared human experience of suffering, sadness, pain, and eventual resolve.

FORGIVENESS

Forgiveness is a process that depending on the situation, usually takes time. Forgiving means letting go of the protective armor of blame and hatred that encases your heart, avoiding putting that person, including yourself, out of your heart. Forgiveness does not mean we suppress our anger, fear, hurt or grief or that we are passive in excusing harmful behavior.

What is helpful on the journey of forgiveness is self-reflection, processing emotions and time. For many of us, including myself, the path of forgiveness has required various forms of support. In addition to a skillful therapist, the ever-present support systems for me have been yoga and meditation practices.

Our most challenging conflicts are usually with the people closest to us. Unfortunately, when both sides hold on to the pain, lack skills in communication and avoid approaching the subject, many important relationships are lost. If one or both sides have the desire to heal their own pain, with proper support and guidance relationships can be recovered. When these relationships continue, there is usually better understanding and more acceptance of the other as well as ourselves.

The interesting discovery about forgiveness is that it gives *you* the most peace rather than the person being forgiven. It's powerful and life changing. We are all humans deserving of love, yet people's actions and behaviors may cause us pain. We can separate the action from the person and wish them well, learn to let go, and ultimately take care of our own well-being.

Incorporating forgiveness in our life is part of our emotional and mental health practices. With the below reflections, notice that forgiveness may have to be towards yourself first. Self-compassion practices can be a useful tool and lay groundwork for forgiveness.

Self-reflection Practice 1

Part 1: Think of a recent situation that was painful and where you may have wished your behavior had been different. Notice if you blame yourself or feel shame around the situation. What are you blaming yourself for? What is the shame about?

Part 2: Keeping this experience in mind, take 5–10 minutes to practice RAIN. (Recognize, Allow, Investigate, Nurture) Make note of your experience. How did the process feel? Do you feel lighter and clearer as a result? This is a practice, so it may take more than one time to settle into the benefits of the practice. Do not rush yourself and make sure to take as much time as needed.

Self-reflection Practice 2

Part 1: Bring self-compassion and support toward yourself and treat yourself as you would want to guide a child, friend or loved one through a difficult situation. Did you speak with yourself as if you were speaking with a loved one? Are you being kind to yourself? Place your hand over your heart and nurture yourself with kind words? Write down your experience.

Part 2: Forgive yourself. Take a moment to notice where you may need to forgive yourself. Tell yourself you forgive you. Be kind and friendly towards yourself. How does that feel? If it's very uncomfortable, imagine speaking to yourself as a young child, or a "future wise self" speaking to you. Write down your experience with self-forgiveness.

_____

_____

_____

_____

_____

_____

_____

_____

_____

Self-reflection Practice 3

Part 1: Recall a recent event *with another person*, that was challenging or something that happened in your past.

Part 2: Bring the same understanding, guidance and support to yourself and *the other person* involved. It helps to place your hand(s) over your heart.

Part 3: Imagine that this person apologized to you for their actions and behaviors that hurt you. Sometimes we may have to imagine the person apologizing, even if it never happens in real life.

_____

_____

_____

_____

_____

Compassion, self-compassion, and forgiveness come from a place of love and result in healing. A consistent practice of yoga and meditation can help lay the groundwork for this healing. A meditation practice or a simple prayer can also be geared towards bringing everyone into our hearts and wishing well for all people around us and throughout the World. The following practice, called a metta meditation, guides us toward being the kind of person we want to be with *our presence* in the world. I recommend practicing some form of metta at the end of a yoga or meditation session.

METTA MEDITATION PRACTICE

The Buddhist metta or loving-kindness meditation, awakens our capacity for unconditional friendliness and love. Our hearts open as we bring our attention to the innate goodness within ourselves and all beings.

1. Sit comfortably in an upright position. Close your eyes and do a scan of the body by letting go of any tension in the shoulders, hands, and belly. Focus on the breath.

2. Bring to your heart someone you love. Take some moments to reflect on the qualities you appreciate most in this person. Send them a loving wish or prayer and even imagine offering a loving embrace.

3. Turn your attention to your own being. Reflect on your own goodness and the goodness of your heart. If it's hard to reflect on your own goodness, recall someone you trust who loves you. You may even imagine yourself as a child or your future wise self.

4. Think of someone you may have a difficult relationship with. It may help to imagine this person as a child or as someone at the end of their life. See if you can look past the hurt and pain and recognize this person's goodness. Imagine offering them a gesture of care, like a warm hug or a kiss on the forehead, or your prayer.

5. Imagine bringing together all the people you just prayed for. Holding yourself and the others in your heart, reflect on your shared humanity and basic goodness.

6. Allow your awareness to open out in all directions. Expand this space of love and care for all beings, all living creatures, and Mother Earth.

7. Rest in the space of silence, awareness, and love.

MONTH 10 CALENDAR

Schedule Yoga Practice 3–5 days per week.

Schedule a 5-minute Meditation 5–7 days per week.

Wellness Calendar

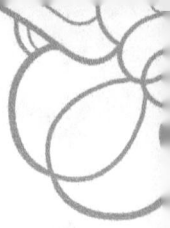

DAY	NIYAMA	ASANA	MEDITATIC
Sunday			
Monday			
Tuesday			
Wednesday			
Thursday			
Friday			
Saturday			

Month 10 _____, Week 1

OBSERVATIONS

Wellness Calendar

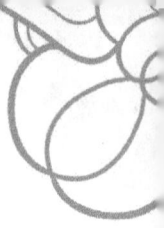

DAY	NIYAMA	ASANA	MEDITATI
Sunday			
Monday			
Tuesday			
Wednesday			
Thursday			
Friday			
Saturday			

Month 10 _____, Week 2

OBSERVATIONS

Wellness Calendar

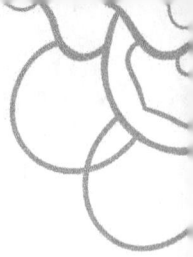

DAY	NIYAMA	ASANA	MEDITATIO
Sunday			
Monday			
Tuesday			
Wednesday			
Thursday			
Friday			
Saturday			

Month 10 _____, Week 3

OBSERVATIONS

Wellness Calendar

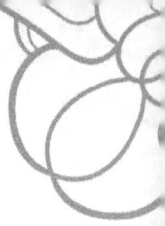

DAY	NIYAMA	ASANA	MEDITATIO
Sunday			
Monday			
Tuesday			
Wednesday			
Thursday			
Friday			
Saturday			

Month 10 _____, Week 4

OBSERVATIONS

Wellness Calendar

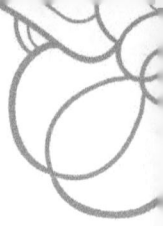

DAY	NIYAMA	ASANA	MEDITATI
Sunday			
Monday			
Tuesday			
Wednesday			
Thursday			
Friday			
Saturday			

Month 10 _____, Week 5

OBSERVATIONS

11
Surrender

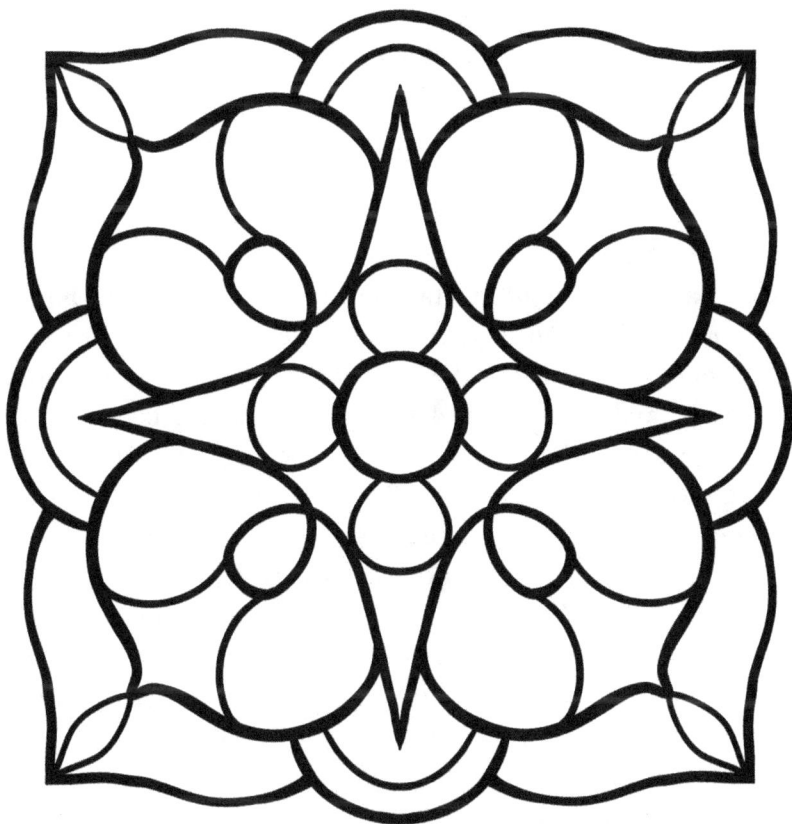

Acceptance and Letting Go

"Wisdom tells me I am nothing. Love tells me I am
everything. And between the two, my life flows."

— *Sri Nisargadatta*

Surrender is a spiritual practice in yoga and meditation. Surrender in meditation is a practice of release as opposed to a practice of control. Mental surrender is a key component in meditation by observing thoughts that come up and learning to let them go. Most people misunderstand meditation as a control practice, yet it is more accurately an act of surrender and liberation. Meditation is not about controlling the mind. It's about surrendering to the fluctuations of the mind while focusing on the flow of the breath. With a consistent connection to the breath, we recognize the thinking mind is what is trying to control.

Surrender during a physical yoga practice is to accept the body for where it is, approach a pose to the best of our ability in that moment, and to let go of mental control and expectations. Further, during meditation and physical yoga practice we may also notice intense emotions come up. We allow them to come, we allow for the release, and we learn to let go. Each practice takes you to a place of surrender. You do your work, whether it be meditation or physical practice, and you let go. The practice of surrender is what ultimately brings you to a place of peace.

To transition from a place of resistance, which is a habit many of us literally "hold on" to, to a place of acceptance is the way to tune into the present moment. Yoga practice emphasizes non- judgment yet acute awareness of *the breath and body. We practice doing our best, accepting the present moment, and letting go or surrendering.*

Meditation and yoga reinforce guiding the mind and body towards restoration and calm. Much of our lives we tend to hold on and try to force or control events and outcomes. As we practice surrender with awareness of our thoughts, our body and breath, we train the brain to do the same in daily life. When we are in the habit of "holding", we are not only tense in the body, but reside in resistance where we hold on to stories, negativity, and fear. Not only does this keep us in fight-or-flight mode, but it keeps us from finding the peace, the home that exists within us.

Self-reflection Journaling 1

Part 1: How often in your day or in your week do you practice *surrender*?

Right now, notice where you are holding tension, and notice where you may be holding a story or event in your mind or body. They may be related. Try letting it go and accept the present moment as it is. Write the thoughts and feelings that may come up. Spend time with it but do not belabor it.

Our ability to surrender mentally, physically, and emotionally is a common practice in our yoga and meditation. It is important to remember that we are not surrendering to the event that causes our suffering — for example, the pain of loss, illness, or death. Instead, we must learn to surrender to **only the present moment**, which is usually not the actual suffering itself. Most often our present moment is exactly that. We may be working at our desks, cleaning, driving or any other activity. The suffering exists mostly in our minds. Each moment is a chance to tune into what is happening now, and **not** what is happening in our minds. The body and the breath are the most accessible ways to root us in the now. Much of our suffering is in the *resisting* rather than in the event itself.

A useful practice is to tune into the breath, tune into sensations like sights and sounds, and tune into the feelings at any given moment. Try asking yourself, "Where am I holding tension in my body at this moment?" Or "How is my breath right now?" Take moments throughout your day to tune in.

Self-Reflection Journaling 2

Recall a challenge you may be having. You may close your eyes, take a moment to scan your body and feel the effects of the challenge in your body. Make note of where you may feel tension such as jaw, shoulders, chest, belly, or lower back. Focus back on your breath. Notice where you are in the *present moment*. Try to stay in this space for 5–10 minutes or more. Write about your experience.

Self-reflection Journaling 3

Part 1: If you make it a life practice to *surrender* to the outcome of events, what does that look like? Do you feel fear or relief, anxiety, or freedom? Do you feel empowered and fearless? Write down your feelings and thoughts.

_____

_____

_____

_____

_____

_____

_____

_____

_____

_____

MONTH 11 CALENDAR

Schedule Yoga Practice 3–5 days per week.

Schedule a 10-minute Meditation 5–7 days per week.

Wellness Calendar

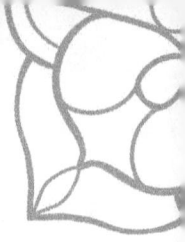

DAY	NIYAMA	ASANA	MEDITATIO
Sunday			
Monday			
Tuesday			
Wednesday			
Thursday			
Friday			
Saturday			

Month 11 _____, Week 1

OBSERVATIONS

Wellness Calendar

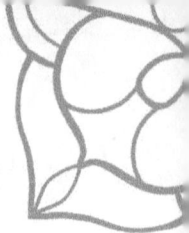

DAY	NIYAMA	ASANA	MEDITATION
Sunday			
Monday			
Tuesday			
Wednesday			
Thursday			
Friday			
Saturday			

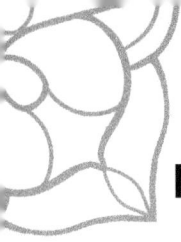

Month 11 _____, Week 2

OBSERVATIONS

Wellness Calendar

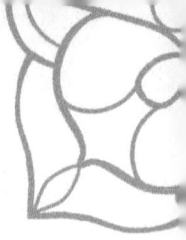

DAY	NIYAMA	ASANA	MEDITATIO
Sunday			
Monday			
Tuesday			
Wednesday			
Thursday			
Friday			
Saturday			

Month 11 _____, Week 3

OBSERVATIONS

Wellness Calendar

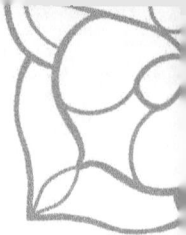

DAY	NIYAMA	ASANA	MEDITATION
Sunday			
Monday			
Tuesday			
Wednesday			
Thursday			
Friday			
Saturday			

Month 11 _____, Week 4

OBSERVATIONS

Wellness Calendar

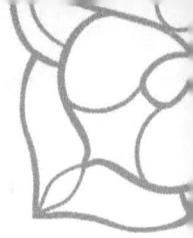

DAY	NIYAMA	ASANA	MEDITATIO
Sunday			
Monday			
Tuesday			
Wednesday			
Thursday			
Friday			
Saturday			

Month 11 _____, Week 5

OBSERVATIONS

Month II   Week 1

12
Your Way Home

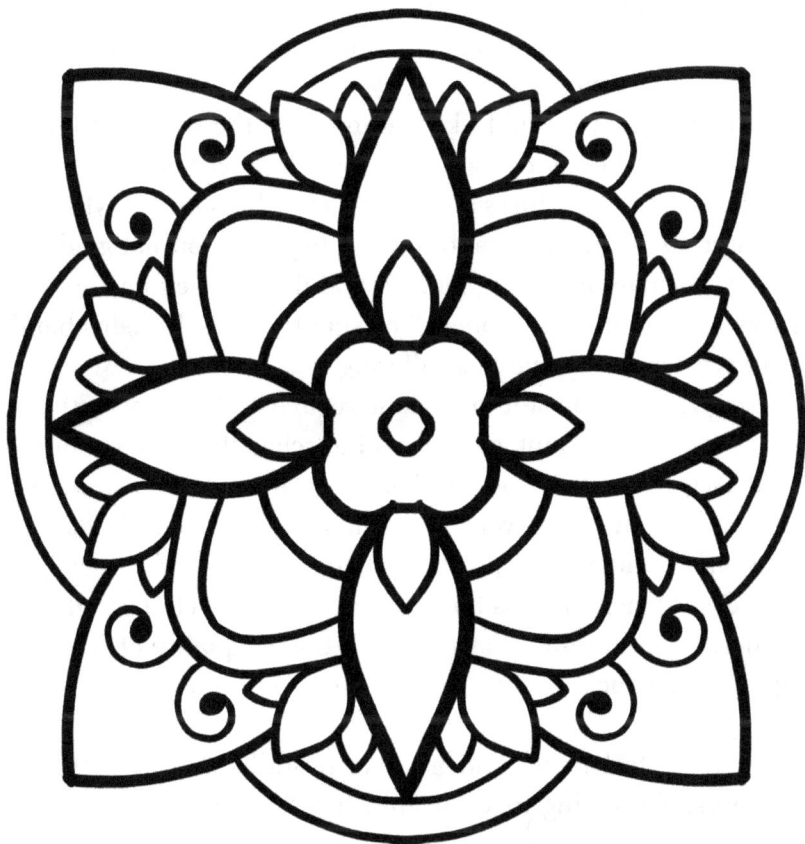

Developing a Personal Practice

"As soon as you honor the present moment,
unhappiness and struggle dissolve,
and life begins to flow with joy and ease."

— *Eckhart Tolle*

The most important aspect of maintaining personal practices is to have a level of enjoyment. When there is enjoyment in an activity, we stick to it. At first, you may find the practices are challenging, and the only enjoyment you experience may be once the practice is over. Remind yourself that as the body and mind become better conditioned, the entire practice — during and after — becomes an enjoyable experience.

In this chapter, I would like you to notice the benefits that consistent yoga, meditation, and self-reflection practices bring to your life. Making these practices a part of your daily routine is where you will discover the most joy and peace. I hope the journal guidelines create a foundation that implements stability and self-healing within yourself and in your "home". The stability in "self "helps build a life of greater clarity and less suffering.

Yoga practice is meant to be done regularly. This is why the calendars are so important, guiding you to schedule and commit each week. To get your 3-day-per-week practice, do not worry necessarily about spacing it out. If your schedule allows for only Friday, Saturday, and Sunday, then practice on those days. Unfortunately for many of us, when life gets busy, the activity to be eliminated is our practice. Keep in mind that to have a higher quality of life, to be "high-performance", our well-being needs to be at the top of our priority list.

When we feel better and have an overall sense of well-being, we are usually taking time for ourselves. This entails taking care of our bodies and more importantly, connecting to ourselves at the deeper levels. I wish for you to continue to practice, maintain your physical, emotional, and mental health, connect to the deeper self, and experience life to its fullest!

In this last month, I encourage you to try a 14-Day Challenge. The challenge encourages daily physical practice that will enhance your experience.

MONTH 12 CALENDAR

It's time to try a
14-Day Challenge!

Schedule a 20–30-minute practice for 14 consecutive days.

Commit to a daily practice and make your yoga mat a space for you "to show up" every day. Remember to be kind to yourself and your body as you practice daily. Approach the challenge as an experiment to self-reflect daily and an opportunity to improve your health.

Wellness Calendar

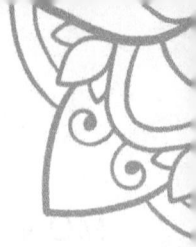

DAY	NIYAMA	ASANA	MEDITATIO
Sunday			
Monday			
Tuesday			
Wednesday			
Thursday			
Friday			
Saturday			

Month 12 _____, Week 1

OBSERVATIONS

Wellness Calendar

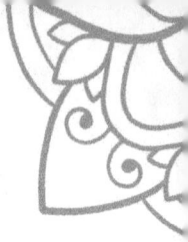

DAY	NIYAMA	ASANA	MEDITATI
Sunday			
Monday			
Tuesday			
Wednesday			
Thursday			
Friday			
Saturday			

Month 12 _____, Week 2

OBSERVATIONS

Wellness Calendar

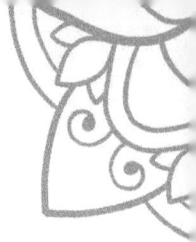

DAY	NIYAMA	ASANA	MEDITATIO
Sunday			
Monday			
Tuesday			
Wednesday			
Thursday			
Friday			
Saturday			

Month 12 _____, Week 3

OBSERVATIONS

Wellness Calendar

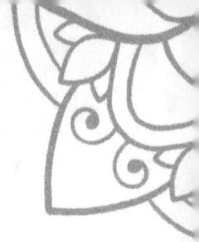

DAY	NIYAMA	ASANA	MEDITATION
Sunday			
Monday			
Tuesday			
Wednesday			
Thursday			
Friday			
Saturday			

Month 12 _____, Week 4

OBSERVATIONS

Wellness Calendar

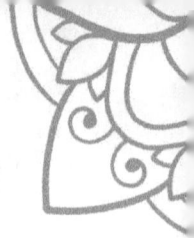

DAY	NIYAMA	ASANA	MEDITATION
Sunday			
Monday			
Tuesday			
Wednesday			
Thursday			
Friday			
Saturday			

Month 12 _____, Week 5

OBSERVATIONS

Self-reflection Journaling 1

How do you feel during your challenge? Do you notice differences in each day's practice? Are you being kind to your body? Are you practicing non-judgement?

Self-reflection Journaling 2

How does it feel to make your physical and mental health a priority for 14 days? Do you feel this challenge is an added pressure or a welcome relief? If this brings up anxiety for you, what part of you is feeling anxious about the challenge? What is the mental messaging?

_____

_____

_____

_____

_____

_____

_____

_____

_____

_____

_____

_____

_____

_____

_____

_____

_____

Self-reflection Journaling 3

Did you notice some habits or patterns of behavior that came up for you?

What *realizations* did this challenge present to you about yourself? About your self-care? About time and energy needed for the challenge? About your mental processes?

_____

_____

_____

_____

_____

_____

CREATING A SAFE SPACE FOR PRACTICE

Yoga is so much more than just another workout. It's an overall approach to better physical, mental, emotional, and spiritual health. Following are some guidelines to help you establish an effective yoga practice.

- Always give it your honest effort. Know that yoga practice may be "uncomfortable," yet it will lead you to improved strength and mobility. The practices will affect your overall well-being on a physical, mental, and emotional level.

- Yoga practice is meant to challenge the body but avoid allowing the ego to take over. The ego is a "mind-made concept" of our identity. Avoid attaching meaning to what your body can and can't do on any particular day. Rather, approach it from a kind and curious observer's perspective.

- Please do not ignore pain sensations. Pain to be avoided is any sensation that may alter the breath. Approach the poses slowly, with care, and awareness of the breath.

- Be aware and mindful of the body each day, and work with the reality of that particular day. The body is different each day, so avoid falling in the trap of expecting the same from your body as it did yesterday, last week or last year.

Closing Thoughts

The highest goal of yoga and meditation practice is to connect deeper within, to connect to consciousness, the Universe, divinity. At first, this may be too much for new practitioners to absorb. What is important with any practice is to be consistent. The beauty of yoga and meditation practice is that benefits occur within the experience of one's own practice. Do not feel you need to subscribe to any belief system, not even in the Eight Limbs of Yoga. When something "rings true" or is understood at the deepest level, it is usually "felt." You experience the *process*, rather than having to believe or disbelieve any writing or concept.

A successful yoga practice is one that makes you feel better at the end of the practice session, one that helps to slow the thinking mind, and helps us tune into the breath.

On some days you may notice that taking a step back in a given pose makes the practice more effective than taking a step forward. The key is to work with the body for *that specific moment* in time. The ego wants more, making us think it's better to move into the next steps, but the body may feel better staying with the integrity of the pose. Wherever you can hold proper alignment of the joints, proper contraction of the muscles, and an even flow or rhythm of breath, is where you maintain the integrity of the pose.

The integrity of a pose is rarely about moving into the more advanced steps. By practicing with full awareness of the body, recognize the foundation lies in the small details. Pay close attention to the *first few steps* of the pose. In addition to re-working the foundational details, you will better understand how to modify most postures in the event of a limitation such as an injury. At some point, we encounter injuries, surgeries and illnesses that will affect our mobility, flexibility, and strength. These hurdles force us to approach postures in a kinder, wiser, and more connected way. Having the proper understanding of the *initial steps* of any pose will help navigate these hurdles with clarity through continued practice.

To conclude, create a space for yourself that is free of distractions. Even if the only uncluttered space is the 2½ by 6-foot space of your yoga mat. Make a commitment to heal the body, to create mobility and strength, or simply to show up for yourself.

This journal includes 4 sequences that incrementally increase the levels of strength and mobility needed. Approach each practice with a "beginner's mind" and stay aware of messages from the body. This practice is *for you*, so remember to use the pose to get into your body as opposed to using your body to get into your pose. Be safe with your practice and enjoy your practice.

Welcome to your path to Finding Home.

www.ingramcontent.com/pod-product-compliance
Lightning Source LLC
Chambersburg PA
CBHW070059030426
42335CB00016B/1944